Employment Issues and Multiple Sclerosis

Employment Issues and Multiple Sclerosis

Phillip D. Rumrill, Jr., Ph.D., CRC
University of Wisconsin—Milwaukee
Department of Educational Psychology

demos vermande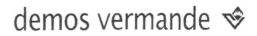

Demos Vermande, 386 Park Avenue South, New York, New York 10016

Library of Congress Cataloging-in-Publication Data

Employment issues and multiple sclerosis / edited by Phillip D.
    Rumrill, Jr.
        p.   cm.
    Includes bibliographical references and index.
    ISBN 1-888799-03-X (pbk.)
    1. Multiple sclerosis—Patients—Employment—United States.
I. Rumrill, Phillip D.
    RC377.E47   1996   96-22536
    331.5'93—dc20   CIP

Made in the United States of America

For Harry, Michele, Stuart, and Douglas

Contents

Preface

Multiple sclerosis (MS) is one of the most common neurologic disorders in the Western Hemisphere. It affects as many as half a million people in the United States alone. Experts in the medical and social sciences have documented the wide-ranging effects that MS exacts on a person's physical, psychological, and social functioning, and virtually every aspect of life has proven susceptible to the illness. The barriers to career development posed by MS often render the illness even more debilitating than the medical symptoms themselves. Although the vast majority of people with MS have employment histories and were working at the time of diagnosis, many are unable to maintain employment as the illness progresses.

This book focuses on the employment issues that inhere to MS. With contributions from nationally prominent authorities in medicine, vocational rehabilitation, and law, chapters consider (1) etiology, incidence, and prevalence; (2) correlates of unemployment; (3) vocational assessment strategies; (4) job placement and retention interventions; (5) the Americans with Disabilities Act; (6) tax benefits and work incentives; and (7) the National Multiple Sclerosis Society's commitment to employment initiatives.

The first four chapters present research-based and somewhat technical descriptions of the medical, psychosocial, and vocational aspects of MS. Specialized terms and professional jargon are defined in the text. With those foundations established, the remaining chapters are devoted to "plain English" discussions of the contemporary employment issues that are most relevant to everyone involved in the American MS community.

Intended for people with MS, their families, physicians, nurses, social workers, rehabilitation professionals, and anyone else interested in the employment implications of MS, *Employment Issues and Multiple Sclerosis* is a resource guide to research, public policy, and service delivery. The text also discusses current trends in health care and rehabilitation and recommends reforms to better serve the interests of people with multiple sclerosis.

Phillip D. Rumrill, Jr., Ph.D.

Acknowledgments

I would like to take this opportunity to thank my friends and colleagues who guided and assisted me in the development of this text. Their expertise was instrumental in the completion of this project.

First, I thank Dr. Diana M. Schneider of Demos Vermande for her editorial consultation, technical assistance, and sponsorship of this book. I hope that this project will represent the first in a long series of collaborative ventures.

For their content-area contributions, I extend sincere gratitude to Ms. Jill Battersby, Ms. Michelle Garnette, Ms. Candace Holman, Ms. Dana Kaleta, and Ms. Jill Steffen of the University of Wisconsin—Milwaukee; free-lance author Mr. Steven Mendelsohn; Mr. Gary Sumner of the National Multiple Sclerosis Society; and Drs. Randall T. Schapiro and Nicholas G. LaRocca for their detailed review of several chapters. Special thanks go to Dr. Richard T. Roessler of the University of Arkansas for his assistance in conceptualizing, composing, and editing the text.

Chapter 1

Etiology, Incidence, and Prevalence

Phillip D. Rumrill, Jr., Dana A. Kaleta, and Jill C. Battersby

Multiple sclerosis (MS) is a degenerative disease of the central nervous system (CNS) characterized by the destruction of the myelin sheath, which insulates white matter tracts in the brain and along the spinal cord. Myelin covering these tracts, or axons, is a fatty tissue that facilitates transmission of electrical impulses to and from the central nervous system. Axons vary in their amount of insulative myelin, but demyelination of any segment of a nerve fiber slows and/or blocks the conveyance of messages throughout the neural chain that sends signals between the brain and the rest of the body via the spinal cord.

Kraft (1981) likened central nervous system demyelination in people with MS to breaks in the rubberized coating that typically surrounds electrical wires. He noted that such breaks interfere with the transmission of electricity, which is precisely what happens in individuals with MS. The result of slowed or blocked neurologic impulses is often observed as uncoordinated and/or awkward responses to environmental stimuli (Wolf, 1984). As patches of myelin deteriorate, they are replaced by scar tissue. The resulting lesions, or plaques, further interrupt the conduction of nerve impulses, creating a progressive and degenerative course of symptoms.

Symptoms associated with MS vary widely depending on the location and size of lesions in the person's brain and spinal cord (Kraft, 1981; Matthews, Cleland, & Hopper, 1970). For example, frontal and parietal lobe lesions often result in cognitive and emotional effects, whereas plaques in the cerebrum, brain stem, and spinal cord tend to cause problems related to the physical

Department of Educational Psychology, University of Wisconsin—Milwaukee functioning of the extremities. Visual impairments may result from direct damage to the optic nerves or the occipital lobe. A significant impediment to fully understanding the etiology of multiple sclerosis lies in the fact that although many people follow a disease course that has certain similarities, no two people with MS experience exactly the same symptoms and course of illness (Gordon, Lewis, & Wong, 1994). Existing research on the physiologic and psychological symptoms of MS is described in greater detail in subsequent sections of this chapter. For additional information concerning the medical aspects of MS, readers are referred to *Symptom Management in Multiple Sclerosis* (Schapiro, 1994), *Multiple Sclerosis and the Family* (Kalb & Scheinberg, eds., 1992), and *Therapeutic Claims in Multiple Sclerosis* (Sibley, 1996).

Causes

Another obstacle to the complete understanding of multiple sclerosis is its elusive origin. Certain groups are more likely to acquire the disease than are others (see "Incidence" and "Prevalence" sections of this chapter), and women are approximately twice as likely to get MS as are men (Kraft, 1981). The precise cause of MS is unknown, but it is thought to be a combination of immunologic, viral, and genetic factors.

Medical scientists have determined that MS involves an autoimmune process; that is, the immune system abnormally directs itself against the central nervous system. Although the exact antigen to which immune cells are directed has not been identified, researchers have discovered which immune cells become sensitized, the process by which they turn on the CNS, and which receptors on the cells are attracted to the myelin sheath.

Epidemiologic studies and migration patterns (National Multiple Sclerosis Society, 1992) show that people who were born in regions where there is a high prevalence of MS and who move to lower prevalence areas acquire the risk of MS of their new homes, provided that the move takes place before the age of fifteen. From these data, some scientists have inferred that there is an environmental agent that activates prior to puberty and predisposes one to develop MS in early or middle adulthood.

Because initial exposure to many viruses occurs during childhood, and because viral factors have been linked to inflammatory responses to demyelination, many experts believe that viral "triggers" catalyze the illness.

Although multiple sclerosis is not hereditary, having a first-degree relative (parent or sibling) who has the illness increases one's risk of acquiring MS by a factor several times that of the risk in the general population (National Multiple Sclerosis Society, 1992). Several studies have also found common genes among certain populations in which there are high rates of MS, but efforts to isolate a single "MS gene" have been unfruitful. Some neurologists have hypothesized that MS develops when a person is genetically susceptible to environmental agents (including viruses) that trigger autoimmune responses. That explanation allows for a reciprocal influence of immunologic, viral, and genetic factors on the development of MS, but its complexity underscores why pinpointing the precise cause of the illness remains an elusive pursuit.

Diagnosis

Until fairly recently, the diagnosis of MS was inferred from presenting symptoms. Because CNS lesions can result from conditions other than MS (e.g., cancer, nutritional deficiencies, traumatic brain injuries), neurologists would necessarily eliminate all other possible causes of lesions before making the diagnosis of MS. Hence, the diagnostic process was often long and laborious. Kraft (1981) noted that an average period of four years intervened between the initial manifestation of MS-related symptoms and diagnosis. Not surprisingly, non- and misdiagnoses were fairly common, and many patients were sent home with a tentative diagnosis of "possible" or "probable" MS to wait for their symptoms to progress before they could receive a definitive diagnosis. Needless to say, the waiting exacted a significant psychological toll on patients and their families (Gordon, Lewis, & Wong, 1994).

Over the past few years, the advent and continued refinement of magnetic resonance imaging (MRI) has enabled neurologists to make an accurate diagnosis of MS in a timely manner, sometimes even before the person evinces any symptoms (Morrissey et al., 1993). In fact, MRI has also shown some promise in predicting the frequency, duration, and intensity of exacerbations of MS following diagnosis (Smith et al., 1994). Even though not all people with MS show abnormalities on MRI scans (Gordon, Lewis, & Wong, 1994; Swanson, 1989), neurologists are able to make the diagnosis of MS with greater speed and accuracy than ever before. MRI has dramatically reduced the time interval between initial symptoms and diagnosis, thereby enabling rehabilitation professionals to initiate early intervention strategies (outlined in Chapter 4) during the preliminary stages of the disease. In turn, early interventions that focus on reasonable accommodations and self-advocacy significantly increase the likelihood that a person with MS will retain his job as the illness progresses (Roessler & Rumrill, 1994b).

Because MRI is not uniformly available and has not yet proven to be a fail-safe predictive tool, medical researchers continue to seek noninvasive and less expensive diagnostic strategies. Whitaker and colleagues (1995) attempted to diagnose MS via myelin-protein analyses in blood and urine, finding a nonsignificant relationship between protein levels and the occurrence of lesions. Nevertheless, they emphasized the need for continued research concerning diagnostic techniques that are both cost-effective and widely available.

Physiologic Effects

The group of physiologic symptoms that has become associated with multiple sclerosis covers a wide range and includes fatigue, mobility problems, spasticity, numbness and tingling in the extremities, general weakness, visual impairments, bowel and bladder dysfunction, and sexual dysfunction. As previously noted, patterns of symptoms have been attributed to the location and size of lesions in the central nervous system.

Any physiologic symptom of MS may be observed in constellation with or in absence of any other(s). When physical symptoms initially occur, they tend to last for several weeks at a time. From that point on, the illness runs a highly unpredictable, often episodic, course. According to Carroll and Dorman (1993, p. 23), "approximately 20 percent of (MS) patients will experience a single attack and never be bothered again. Ten percent will experience symptoms that become permanent and quickly progress, sometimes to the point of incapacitation. The remaining 70 percent will have symptoms that appear, disappear, then reappear again at varying intervals of time and degrees of severity."

The wide range of physical symptoms and the capricious disease process pose significant impediments for people with MS in virtually every aspect of personal and social functioning. To the extent that work is an all too frequent casualty of MS, rehabilitation professionals and people with MS alike must view the symptoms described in the following paragraphs in light of their potential impact on employment and other life activities.

Fatigue

The most common effect of MS is unquestionably fatigue (Kraft, 1981). Although it does not always present itself as a single, easily identifiable symptom, fatigue affects people with MS in several specific ways. Schapiro (1994) identified four distinct types of fatigue that are commonly observed in people with MS: normal fatigue, fatigue of depression, fatigue of "short-circuiting," and MS fatigue or lassitude. Each has unique signs and implications for self-care.

Normal Fatigue

The first and least invasive form of fatigue is a persistent, general tiredness similar to that experienced at the end of a hard day of work (Schapiro, 1994). For most people who do not have MS, it is a normal condition that can be accommodated quite simply by a good night's sleep.

Depression-Related Fatigue

A more intrusive form of MS-related fatigue is characterized by feeling "worn-out." This often affects the person's sleep pattern and appetite, and it manifests in a sense of listlessness, apathy, and diminished self-esteem. These subsymptoms mirror those associated with depression, and they are hence treated most effectively with antidepressant medication and/or psychotherapy. Accordingly, Sibley (1996) labeled "worn-out" fatigue a psychological condition.

"Short-Circuiting"

According to Schapiro (1994), "short-circuiting" fatigue results from physically overtaxing oneself. Hardening and scarring of the myelin sheath along neural pathways lead to a reduction in the smooth transmission of electrical impulses to the extremities. This inefficiency results in the slowing and eventual stoppage of physical activity until the person with MS has rested and regained his or her energy. Unlike depression-related fatigue, short-circuiting fatigue is primarily physiologic in nature (Sibley, 1996).

MS Fatigue

The fourth type of fatigue described by Schapiro (1994) is termed "MS fatigue" because it seems to be unique to people coping with the illness. MS fatigue is typified by an overwhelming sense of exhaustion that affects the individual suddenly and without warning. These bouts of complete fatigue may last for a few hours or for several days. They may also end as suddenly as they began, leaving the person with what seems to be a "burst" of energy. The only proven antidotes for MS fatigue are sleep and time.

Generally, all four types of fatigue that are commonly reported by people with MS are exacerbated by stress and by an increase in body temperature. Because exercise, being outside in hot weather, and taking hot baths have been shown to increase fatigue in people with MS, these activities should be monitored or avoided whenever possible. A stress management regimen has also proven to be an effective means of controlling fatigue and allowing the person with MS to conserve energy for necessary daily living activities.

Motor Disturbances

A number of physiologic symptoms are related to motor disturbances in people with MS, including spasticity, weakness, and ataxia. These lead to general coordination, balance, and mobility impairments (Kraft, 1981). The extent and type of these effects vary widely among (and even within) people with MS, but motor disturbances are typically among the first manifestations of the illness.

Spasticity

Spasticity is a disruption in the coordination of muscle contraction and relaxation. This is a common symptom of MS because of damage in the descending motor pathways that carry impulses from the spinal cord to control muscular reflexes. When lesions occur along these pathways, they cause opposite muscles within a group to contract and relax simultaneously, or spasm. Spasms are most common in the legs (flexor and extensor muscles), and people with MS most frequently experience spasticity at night (Matthews, 1985).

Weakness

MS is often characterized by a loss of strength in major muscle groups such as those of the arms and legs. Schapiro (1994) noted that observed weakness in people with MS more often results from poorly transmitted neural impulses than from deterioration of the muscles themselves. However, misconduction of impulses makes it difficult for the person with MS to fully utilize the affected muscles, and prolonged underutilization can cause the muscles to atrophy.

Backaches are a common secondary symptom of MS, most often attributed to strain resulting from compensation for weakness and fatigue in the legs (Matthews, 1985).

Ataxia

The inability to move the arms or walk in a coordinated fashion is another frequently observed effect of MS-related weakness. In combating muscular weakness, priority must be placed on conserving energy for activities of daily living and symptom management. Because some exercises exacerbate muscle weakness and fatigue, people with MS should always consult their physicians and/or physical therapists before initiating a conditioning program.

Ambulation, the simple act of walking and getting around, is often impaired by such symptoms as balance problems, hyperextension of the knees, and instability of the legs. A condition called "foot drop" (Schapiro, 1994), in which toes touch the ground prior to the heel strike, adds to instability and ambulatory difficulties. Orthotic devices such as stabilizing braces and plastic shoe inserts may improve gait problems and aid in ambulation by controlling foot drop and hyperextension.

Numbness and Tingling

Numbness and tingling in the extremities can range from "pins and needles" to itching in an isolated area of skin or a more severe and painful condition called trigeminal neuralgia (Matthews, 1985). Pins and needles down the back and legs may occur when one bends his or her neck. Although not painful, the sensation can be bothersome. Trigeminal neuralgia involves the onset of sudden, sharp pain in one side of the face. It results from the discharge of impulses from the brain stem. The accompanying pain typically lasts for only ten to fifteen seconds, but it is characteristically followed by a facial contraction, or tic (Matthews, 1985).

Tremor

Tremor in the extremities and head is another common physiologic symptom of MS, manifested in a wide range of movement from fine, less noticeable tremors to gross, more obvious oscillations (Schapiro, 1994).

Visual Impairments

Visual impairments in people with MS are most often temporary conditions that manifest in blurred or double vision, although in some cases functional blindness may result. They result from optic neuritis (inflammation of the optic nerve) and are frequently marked by dulled color vision, diminished visual acuity, and a reduced visual field (Schapiro, 1994). Optic neuritis is one of the most common early symptoms of MS (Johnson & Johnson, 1978), and it is often indicative of a more benign form of the illness. Other MS-related visual impairments result from weakening of the eye muscle and nystagmus (eye jerking).

Bowel and Bladder Dysfunction

Bowel and bladder dysfunctions are frequent, frustrating, and often embarrassing effects of MS. These difficulties include urgency, dribbling, hesitancy, frequency, and incontinence. Bowel and bladder dysfunctions can have a negative impact on a person's daily living regimen, but they can often be effectively managed through medication and/or diet.

Sexual Dysfunction

Although it is not directly related to work and career development, the issue of sexual dysfunction in people with multiple sclerosis requires consideration within the context of general symptomatology. The effects of sexual dysfunction can be pervasive, often manifesting in psychological and family problems in addition to their physiologic accompaniments. Often associated with fatigue, specific sexual problems frequently encountered by people with MS include retarded and premature ejaculation, decreased vaginal and penile sensation, impotence, vaginal dryness, anorgasmia, decreased sex drive, and slowed response and arousal time (Barrett, 1984).

Course and Progression

The unpredictable course of multiple sclerosis is one of the most difficult aspects of the illness. Specifically, the nature, severity, and number of MS-related symptoms vary widely among individuals. Moreover, the patterns that mark symptom manifestation, typically in terms of relapses and remissions, cannot be generalized from one person to the next. These patterns have, however, been codified to provide a clearer understanding of the different "types" of MS that people experience. Gross and Sinaki (1987) identified four general courses of MS: (1) benign, (2) relapsing-remitting, (3) chronic progressive, and (4) malignant. The following paragraphs describe the characteristic pattern of each course.

Benign MS

The benign form of multiple sclerosis is marked by long periods of remission, arrested symptom manifestation, and relative stability of health between relapses of the illness. Initial symptoms occur suddenly and without warning, but they generally do not increase in severity with each successive relapse. Exacerbations may involve recurrence of initial symptoms and/or the introduction of symptoms that the person has not previously experienced (Gross & Sinaki, 1987), but the benign course of MS tends to be relatively unintrusive compared to other forms of the illness.

The most benign form of MS involves a single incident of symptoms followed by a permanent state of remission. Approximately 20 percent of people diagnosed with MS experience this "one time" course (Carroll & Dorman, 1993).

Although physicians are as yet unable to predict the course of MS in a given patient with any real certainty, some inferences can be made when certain initial symptoms appear in the absence of others. For example, when visual impairment resulting from damage to the optic nerve occurs in isolation as a person's first symptom, he or she can generally expect a more benign course of MS than can a person whose initial symptoms are physiologic in nature, such as motor disturbances (Matthews, 1985). Schapiro (1994) suggested a fifth category, benign sensory MS, to include people whose illness is marked by isolated and nonprogressive visual impairment.

Relapsing-Remitting MS

Gross and Sinaki (1987) described relapsing-remitting MS as a course in which exacerbations of the illness typically occur several months apart. Accompanied by any number of symptoms, these episodic relapses may persist for a period of several years or over the course of a lifetime. Moreover, each successive exacerbation tends to be increasingly severe and longer lasting, and recovery becomes more difficult. However, remissions do tend to return the person to a baseline level of functioning that is fairly stable over time (Schapiro, 1994). In other words, although relapsing-remitting MS is marked by progressively intrusive exacerbations, the illness is usually rendered benign during remissions.

Chronic Progressive MS

Although MS is widely viewed as an episodic illness marked by cycles of relapses and remissions, many people experience a slow, steadily progressive trail of symptoms that results in increased functional decrements over time. Chronic progressive MS can include any or all of the physiologic symptoms described in this chapter, the most common being fatigue, weakness, and mobility problems (Gross & Sinaki, 1987). People with this type of MS also tend to be less responsive to chemotherapies than are those with relapsing-remitting MS.

Malignant MS

A small minority of people with MS experience an aggressive, persistent, and life-threatening form of the illness. According to Gross and Sinaki (1987), malignant MS is characterized by an intense incident of initial symptoms followed by a short and precipitous progression that renders the person incapacitated. Malignant MS is a rare, terminal form of the illness, for which there is no known treatment.

Psychological Effects

As if the physiologic accompaniments of multiple sclerosis were not debilitating enough, the illness often has a negative impact on psychological functioning. Psychological problems related to MS can be divided into three categories: (1) cognitive dysfunction, (2) affective disorders, and (3) adjustmental issues.

Cognitive Dysfunction

Although once considered symptomatic of only the most severe cases of MS, cognitive dysfunction has been established as a common symptom of all stages and types of the disease (Rao, 1986). Peyser, Rao, LaRocca, and Kaplan (1990) estimated that as many as 65 percent of those diagnosed with MS experience some degree of cognitive dysfunction. Because MS can destroy myelin anywhere in the CNS, its associated cognitive impairments cover the gamut, including memory disturbances and reasoning deficits. These effects tend to be specific to the location of associated lesions; MS does not typically precipitate a decline in general intellectual ability (Peyser et al., 1990).

In terms of memory disturbance, Rao, Leo, and St. Aubin-Faubert (1989) found that people with MS exhibited deficits on measures of long-term memory and verbal fluency. However, participants performed normally on measures of short-term memory, immediate memory (recognition), and rate of forgetting from long-term memory. The authors concluded that memory disturbance in MS results primarily from an impaired ability to access information from long-term memory, whereas encoding and storage capacities remain intact. They also noted that the degree of memory disturbance in their sample was not related to duration of illness (length of time since diagnosis) or severity of physical disability.

In another study on memory disturbance in MS, Grant and colleagues (1984) reported significant decrements in short-term memory, the ability to learn new information, and the ability to retrieve learned information. They also found people with MS to be more susceptible to proactive interference (distraction) during memory recall tasks than a comparison group of people who did not have MS.

Numerous other cognitive impairments have been linked to lesions in the frontal lobe. McIntosh-Michaelis and colleagues (1991) found that approximately one-third of a sample of MS patients exhibited frontal lobe damage, manifested in such symptoms as behavior and personality changes, poor functioning in social roles, diminished planning abilities, and reduced insight and empathy.

Affective Disorders

A sizable portion of the overall psychological impact of MS can be viewed in terms of affective disorders that have been shown to accompany the illness. Foremost among these is depression. Minden, Orav, and Reich (1987) reported that more than half (54 percent) of a sample of people with MS had experienced at least one major depressive episode since the onset of their illness. More recently, findings presented by Minden and Schiffer (1990) upheld the approximately 50 percent prevalence rate of depression among individuals with MS. Although existing studies have established depression as a major psychological symptom of MS, it has yet to be determined whether depressive episodes result from neurologic abnormalities or manifest as a psychological response to a serious illness.

Specifically, Minden, Orav, and Reich (1987) described the typical depressive episodes experienced by people with MS as moderately severe and marked by anger, irritability, worry, and discouragement rather than self-criticism and/or withdrawal. People with MS who experienced depression most frequently were those who had reported depression prior to the onset of MS and those who had received the steroid prednisone to treat acute exacerbations of the illness (Minden, Orav, & Reich, 1987).

In addition to clinical depression, people with MS evidence higher rates of bipolar affective disorder than does the general population (Minden & Schiffer, 1990). Bipolar disorder is characterized by cyclical patterns of severe depression interspersed with periods of mania and/or euphoria.

Euphoria, a persistent feeling of well-being and optimism in spite of negative circumstances, is sometimes exhibited by people with MS in isolation of other symptoms (Rao, Huber, & Bornstein, 1992). Minden and Schiffer (1990, p. 98) stated that "euphoria in MS is not a fluctuating emotional state or a reversible mood but rather a persistent frame of mind and outlook, an apparent and permanent change in personality."

Another occasional psychological symptom of multiple sclerosis is pathological laughing and weeping. A person with MS may break into laughter or begin weeping with slight provocation, regardless of the underlying mood state (Minden & Schiffer, 1990). Such emotional outbursts can be functionally disabling in and of themselves, making even rudimentary tasks of daily living extremely difficult.

Psychological Adjustment

In addition to the cognitive and affective symptoms of MS, the wide-ranging physiologic effects of the illness and its capricious course make the process of adjusting to such a debilitating disease a very difficult task. To the extent that MS often renders the person more dependent on others than he was prior to onset of the illness, friends, family, and colleagues are an integral aspect of the process of adjustment.

Matson and Brooks (1977) created a psychological adjustment model pertaining specifically to people with MS. The model describes the interpersonal and intrapersonal changes that people experience as they learn to cope with the illness. The developmental model of Matson and Brooks includes four stages: denial, resistance, affirmation, and integration. They are operationalized in the following paragraphs.

Denial

According to Matson and Brooks, people with MS typically go through an initial period of denial immediately after learning of their diagnosis. In the denial stage, the person often challenges her diagnosis, seeks alternative medical opinions, attempts to hide symptoms from others, refuses help, and endeavors to live as she did before onset of the illness. Denial is intended to give the appearance that "everything is normal" in the person's life, but it results in such nonnormative effects as withdrawal from family and friends and social isolation.

Resistance

In the second stage, resistance, the person with MS spends a great deal of time and energy searching for cures or treatments to combat the illness. Still reluctant to accept help from others, the person begins to realize the personal and social changes that impend as he continues to cope with MS. During the resistance stage, many people with MS join self-help groups, initiate physical therapy and/or exercise programs, and establish active self-care regimens in an effort to minimize the effects of the illness.

Affirmation

Affirmation, the third stage of adjustment to MS, begins when the person acknowledges the illness and takes steps toward accepting the life changes that became evident during the stage of resistance. Common emotional reactions during this stage include grief over the perceived loss of one's former self, fear of future decrements in functioning, and anxiety or uncertainty concerning what will happen next (Marsh, Ellison, & Strite, 1983). On a more positive note, people in the affirmation stage begin to accept help from others and settle into realistic treatment regimens.

Integration

The fourth and final stage, integration, occurs when the person with MS learns to live with the disease on a day-by-day basis. No longer preoccupied with issues of disability or health, he "integrates" effective coping responses with assistance from family and friends. Obviously, complete acceptance of MS is difficult to achieve. Not everyone reaches the final stage of adjustment, and exacerbations of the illness can impede one's ability to make integrated coping responses.

A number of factors influence one's progression through the stages of adjustment to MS. A primary determinant of adjustment is the overall intrusiveness of the illness—that is, the cumulative effect of (1) functional deficits, physical disabilities, and stressful life events (Devins et al., 1993); (2) the unique constellation of signs, symptoms, and treatment constraints associated with an individual's condition (Devins et al., 1993); (3) disease activity, life-satisfaction, coping style, and knowledge of MS (Devins & Seland, 1987); and (4) personality and social support systems (Burnfield & Burnfield, 1982). This list clearly reflects the individual and often unpredictable nature of adjustment to MS.

The far-reaching psychological accompaniments of MS solidify its designation as one of the most difficult diseases to cope with, adjust to, and, ultimately, accept (Rumrill, 1993). The nature and progression of physiologic and neurologic symptoms exact a significant toll on those diagnosed with MS as well as on their families and friends, and the adjustmental and social issues that inhere to MS remain among the most difficult effects of the illness to treat.

Treatment

Just as no certainty exists as to the cause of MS, no treatment modality has been reliably demonstrated to prevent onset of the illness, progression of CNS lesions, or development of new lesions. Moreover, no medical procedure—surgical, chemotherapeutic, or otherwise—has been developed to alter or dissipate existing lesions. However, adrenocorticotropic hormones and corticosteroids (prednisone) have been shown to reduce the severity of exacerbations among some people with MS (Kraft, 1981). Such treatments as a fat-free diet, sunflower oil, and vitamin supplements have not proven efficacious.

According to Waksman, Reingold, and Reynolds (1987, p. 81), "the characteristic fluctuating course of MS means that most patients' bodies have the innate capacity to terminate an exacerbation and to maintain a remission for relatively long periods of time." Hence, most MS treatments have been oriented toward catalyzing the body's own immune responses to neurologic irregularities. One of the problems in evaluating the efficacy of such treatments is that it is impossible to determine whether an improvement or remission is a result of the treatment or of the natural course of the illness.

Physicians have the ability to specify MS treatment regimens to an individual's course and symptoms (Schapiro, 1990), but the search continues for curative treatments that will prevent or arrest the underlying agents of the disease. To that end, several medications have shown recent promise in experimental and limited-use applications in extending remissions and deintensifying exacerbations of MS. These include Betaseron® (interferon beta-1b), Avonex® (interferon beta-1a), Copaxone® (copolymer-1), Myloral® (oral myelin), and Leustatin® (cladribine) (National Multiple Sclerosis Society, 1995).

Incidence and Prevalence

Although medical historians speculate that early versions of multiple sclerosis date back as many as six hundred years, the disease was not named until 1868, when the French clinician Charcot labeled it "sclérose en plaques." Charcot is credited as the first scientist to link the symptoms of MS to demyelination and lesions in the central nervous system (Waksman, Reingold, & Reynolds, 1987).

A little more than a century later, MS is firmly established as one of the most common neurologic disorders in the Western Hemisphere. The National Multiple Sclerosis Society estimates the prevalence of MS in the United States to be between 250,000 and

350,000 cases (Reingold, 1995). In a recent worldwide study, Dean (1994) estimated that approximately 1,080,000 people across the globe have MS (20.6 cases per 100,000 people).

Although MS can occur at any age, initial manifestations are most often evident during early adulthood, typically between the ages of twenty and forty years (Reingold, 1995). In fact, half of the diagnoses of MS are conferred before a person's thirtieth birthday, and three-quarters of Americans with MS were diagnosed before the age of forty (Waksman, Reingold, & Reynolds, 1987).

Multiple sclerosis is much more common among women than men. Estimates of women:men ratios within the American MS community have ranged from 1.5:1 (Matthews, 1985) to 2:1 (Reingold, 1995). The prevalence of MS also varies markedly according to geography. Epidemiologic studies have revealed higher prevalence rates in temperate regions than in warmer climates. Countries that have particularly high rates of MS include the United Kingdom, Canada, Germany, Scandinavian countries, and the United States. Within the United States, Baum and Rothschild (1981) cited the 37th Parallel (which divides the American population roughly in half) as a geographic demarcation that separates areas marked by high and low risks for MS. They found that Americans residing north of the 37th Parallel were nearly twice as likely to have MS as those in the southernmost half of the population.

To the extent that people living in countries in which MS is most common are predominantly white, the incidence and prevalence of MS vary significantly along racial lines. Poser (1987) pointed out that MS is extremely uncommon in Asian peoples, unknown in African blacks, and relatively infrequent in African-Americans. He also noted that people of Hispanic descent are far less likely to develop MS than those of Germanic, Anglo-Saxon, and Scandinavian lineages.

Summary

Multiple sclerosis is one of the most prevalent neurologic disorders in the United States. Characterized by an unpredictable course, the illness destroys white matter tracts in the central nervous system. Depending on where the nerve damage occurs, people with MS evince a wide range of physiologic and psychological symptoms, including fatigue, mobility problems, spasticity, numbness and tingling in the extremities, general weakness, visual impairments, bowel and bladder dysfunction, sexual dysfunction, cognitive disabilities, depression, anxiety, and diminished self-efficacy.

Diagnosing multiple sclerosis has become much easier in recent years with the advent of magnetic resonance imaging, but the medical community has been unable as yet to determine the underlying cause of the disease. Most conventional theories concerning the origin of MS espouse an interaction among immunologic, viral, and genetic factors as the most plausible cause, but attempts to specify that interaction have been inconclusive.

There is presently no cure for MS, but certain recent chemotherapeutic regimens have shown encouraging success in extending the duration of remissions and deintensifying exacerbations of the illness. More research is needed to develop treatments that impede and arrest the progression of this often devastating disease.

Prevalence rates vary widely along gender, cultural, and geographic lines. Women are about twice as likely as men to develop MS, and the illness predominates among individuals of white, northern European descent. The geographic distribution of MS is also worth noting; two-thirds of the American MS population reside in the northernmost 50 percent of the population.

Multiple sclerosis is distinct from other diseases in course, range of symptoms, and populational demography. It also has a unique, often deleterious impact on personal and social functioning. To the extent that a person's work role constitutes an important element of personal and social functioning, the impact of MS on career development is an important consideration for health care providers, rehabilitation professionals, and people with MS and their families. The following chapters provide a comprehensive overview of the work-related issues that people with MS encounter as they cope with this intrusive disease.

Chapter 2

Correlates of Unemployment

Phillip D. Rumrill, Jr.

Given the range and severity of symptoms associated with multiple sclerosis, it should be of little surprise that the disease can deleteriously affect virtually every aspect of personal and social functioning. As the illness progresses and the symptoms become increasingly frequent and intense, the person often finds himself unable to perform tasks of daily living in the same manner as prior to the onset of the illness.

One life role that is often interrupted by MS is work. In the United States and many industrialized countries, who we are is determined in large measure by what we do for a living (Zunker, 1994). When we are introduced to strangers at social functions, one of the first items of information we share is our occupation. In fact, we tend to describe our jobs as defining attributes of our being—"I'm an architect." Work consumes a considerable portion of a person's identity, and its influence begins early in childhood and continues throughout the life cycle (Super, 1980).

Consider, then, the potentially devastating impact of MS on an individual's career and personal development. As noted in the previous chapter, the onset of MS typically occurs between the ages of twenty and forty years, a time that many people regard as the "prime of life." From the standpoint of career development, those years are the most active decades of most people's lives. According to Super (1980), the period between ages twenty and forty is marked by (1) exploration (gathering and processing occupational information to formulate career goals); (2) establishment (forging a plan for attainment of those goals and beginning a career); and (3) maintenance activities (advancing in one's career and attaining goals). For many people with MS, however, the career development process slows and, in many cases, stops after the illness manifests itself.

More than 90 percent of Americans with MS have employment histories; that is, they have worked in the past (LaRocca, 1995). Some 60 percent were employed at the time of diagnosis, even given the extended time period that until recently typically intervened between initial symptom manifestation and confirmed diagnosis. As time and the illness progress, however, people with MS experience a precipitous decline in employment. LaRocca (1995) reported that only about 25 percent of Americans with MS were employed at the time of this writing. Numerous researchers in the medical and social sciences have attempted to explain the low rate of employment among people with MS, and this chapter examines the factors that contribute to job retention and loss. To that end, I review research on correlates of unemployment such as (1) demographic characteristics, (2) physiologic symptoms, (3) cognitive dysfunction, (4) psychological factors, (5) workplace variables, (6) work disincentives in the Social Security program, and (7) health insurance issues.

Demographic Characteristics

For the general population, as well as for people with MS, prospects of job tenure and career success are often subject to demographic influences. Demographic factors that have been linked to employment status in MS research include gender, socioeconomic status, and age.

Gender

Gender is foremost among the demographic correlates of unemployment for people with multiple sclerosis. Although the unemployment rate among Americans with MS is disappointingly high for both sexes, women are significantly less likely to be employed than men (LaRocca, 1995; LaRocca & Holland, 1982). In 1985, LaRocca, Kalb, Scheinberg, and Kendall reported that 80 percent of New York City area women with MS were unemployed, as compared to 66 percent of men with the illness. These figures are especially troubling when viewed in light of the comparatively low rates of unemployment reported by a reference group of nondisabled men (19 percent) and women (50 percent). A larger national survey one year later revealed unemployment rates of 84 percent and 72 percent, respectively, for women and men with MS (Kornblith, LaRocca, & Baum, 1986). Canadians with MS appear to experience similar gender disparities; Edgley, Sullivan, and Dehoux (1991) reported unemployment rates of 58 percent and 70 percent for men and women, respectively.

Moreover, other correlates of unemployment seem to affect people with MS differently across gender lines. For example, mobility impairment is a strong predictor of job loss for men, whereas women tend to leave the workforce before they evince severe physical symptoms (Kornblith, LaRocca, & Baum, 1986). Also, a lower level of educational attainment was associated with unemployment among men with MS but not among women (Kornblith, LaRocca, & Baum, 1986).

Socioeconomic Status

Although marital status is not related to employment status (LaRocca et al., 1985), both men and women with MS are more likely to leave the workforce if they have a spouse who is working (Genevie, Kallos, & Struenig, 1987). People with MS who have higher levels of education and/or more money in savings and investments are more likely to be employed than are those in lower socioeconomic strata (Edgley, Sullivan, & Dehoux, 1991; Genevie, Kallos, & Struenig, 1987). Genevie, Kallos, and Struenig explained this finding by suggesting that people with higher levels of education tend to occupy positions that require less physical exertion, and that the physiologic effects of MS therefore do not impose work handicaps to the same extent as they do for those whose jobs require more exertion. They also noted that higher-level employees have more flexibility and autonomy in "tailoring" their jobs to meet MS-related needs. Indeed, employers are generally more likely to accommodate workers who are viewed as talented and essential to the operation of business than they are to meet the needs of less valued workers (Rumrill, 1993).

Even so, LaRocca (1995) suggested that many people with MS who have the financial means to stop working do so voluntarily, and Duggan, Fagan, and Yateman (1993) reported that three-quarters of unemployed people with MS had left the workforce of their own volition. Those who leave the workforce are unlikely to return; LaRocca (1995) estimated that only one-third of unemployed Americans with MS were interested in resuming their careers.

Age

In an Israeli study, Rozin, Schiff, Kahana, and Soffer (1975) found that age played a role in unemployment among people with MS, with older workers tending to leave their jobs at a higher rate than younger ones. In a survey of 1,180 Canadians with MS, Edgley, Sullivan, and Dehoux (1991) found unemployment to increase as a direct function of age.

Respondents between the ages of 20 and 29 reported a 38 percent jobless rate, a significantly lower proportion than those rates indicated by their counterparts at ages 30–39 (57 percent), 40–49 (70 percent), 50–59 (84 percent), 60–69 (87 percent), and 70 and over (93 percent). However, only 6 percent of the individuals queried actually responded, and these percentages may not be generalizable to the entire MS community.

The relationship between age and unemployment in people with MS has been upheld in several studies in the United States (Genevie, Kallos, & Struenig, 1987; Kornblith, LaRocca, & Baum, 1986). LaRocca, Kalb, Scheinberg, and Kendall (1985) presented findings indicating a curvilinear direction of that relationship; they found middle-aged people with MS more likely to be employed than either younger or older people.

Two factors related to MS and unemployment might help to explain why seasoned, older workers tend to leave the workforce before reaching retirement age. First, there is a significant relationship between age and MS-related functional disability (Wineman, 1990); as the years pass and the illness progresses, the person becomes less able to meet the physical demands of employment. Second, age is positively associated with socioeconomic status; many older people with MS have the financial means to stop working and do so voluntarily to focus on other pursuits (Keniston, 1995).

Demographic Characteristics for Future Inquiry: Race and Population Density

The current literature contains reports of several well-conducted studies concerning the demographic characteristics associated with unemployment among people with multiple sclerosis, but further inquiry is needed to specify who leaves the workforce, under what circumstances they stop working, and what factors influence their decisions. In concluding their study, Rozin, Schiff, Kahana, and Soffer (1975, p. 303) wrote, "no significant factor was found to explain the reasons why patients (with MS) with working potential are unemployed. Their educational background, work history, vocational education and demographic data supply no clues." Indeed, the next step appears to warrant causal comparative approaches to identify the demographic factors that underlie the high rate of unemployment among people with MS.

One demographic variable that seems to have been given insufficient attention to date is that of racial and ethnic identity. Although the majority of Americans with MS are of northern European descent, enough people of color have been diagnosed with the illness to consider whether the cultural and economic disadvantages associated with minority status in the United States have an impact on employment. Also, does *where* one lives have anything to do with employment prospects when coping with MS? Cross-disability research indicates that limited job options and poor access to transportation place people with disabilities who reside in rural areas at a disadvantage when it comes to employment, whereas their urban counterparts find it easier to choose, obtain, and travel to their jobs (Rubin & Roessler, 1995). Research with cross-sectional national samples would shed light on the extent to which these and other demographic factors have an impact on employment.

Physiologic Symptoms

Researchers have reported mixed results concerning the impact of specific physiologic symptoms of MS on employment, but in general researchers have found the exacerbation and progression of physical effects of the illness to be a strong predictor of job loss.

Physical Limitations and Fatigue

In delineating the most commonly voiced reasons that people with MS leave the workforce, LaRocca, Kalb, Scheinberg, and Kendall

(1985) cited physical limitations as the most frequently given (27.5 percent). Fatigue (13.9 percent) and visual impairment (7.4 percent) were other symptom-related factors that correlated with unemployment. More specifically, a participant's score on the Kurtzke Disability Status Scale (a measure for determining severity of physical disability based on neurologic examination and functional assessment) was indicated as a significant predictor of employment status—the more severe the physical disability, the more likely a participant was to be unemployed (LaRocca et al., 1985). Gulick, Yam, and Touw (1989) found ambulatory (walking) problems to be associated with unemployment, as did Kornblith, LaRocca, and Baum (1986).

Consistent with these findings, Genevie, Kallos, and Struenig (1987) showed significant relationships between unemployment and such symptoms as numbness/tingling, speech problems, visual impairments, pain, fatigue, motor disturbances, and ambulatory problems. In summarizing their findings, Edgley, Sullivan, and Dehoux (1991, p. 131) wrote, "ambulation difficulties and fatigue are the most frequently reported causes of unemployment in individuals with MS." Approximately 41 percent of unemployed respondents in the survey reported by Edgley, Sullivan, and Dehoux cited ambulatory difficulties as the primary reason for their discontinuation of employment. Thirty-nine percent described fatigue as the most important contributing factor. To a lesser extent, visual impairment, loss of coordination, pain, and incontinence were also noted.

On the contrary, Gregory, Disler, and Firth (1993) found no relationship between mobility problems and unemployment among people with MS in New Zealand. They suggested that improvements in assistive technology over the past several years have mitigated the effects of the physiologic symptoms of MS on personal and social functioning. They did cite the inability to work a full day as a common barrier, but they attributed that difficulty to fatigue and a resultant lack of concentration rather than to mobility problems.

Disease-Related Factors: Age at Onset, Duration of Illness, and Course

Apart from the physiologic symptoms, Gordon, Lewis, and Wong (1994, p. 34) noted, "vocational planning for people with MS is complicated due to the progressive and unpredictable nature of the disorder." Indeed, the age at which one was diagnosed with MS (Mitchell, 1981) and the duration and course of the disease (Bauer, Firnhaber, & Winkler, 1965) have also been associated with unemployment. Bauer, Firnhaber, and Winkler (1965) found that those with chronic symptom progression from onset were the least likely to be employed, followed, respectively, by people with exacerbating/progressive symptoms and individuals whose illness was marked by episodic exacerbations and remissions.

The wide range of physical symptoms that results from demyelination in the central nervous system has been shown to impede people with MS in virtually every life role. Moreover, the often episodic and progressive course of the illness makes it doubly difficult to anticipate and cope with MS-related symptoms. Consequently, the energies that were expended on work and leisure activities are often consumed by symptom management. Advancements in assistive and adaptive technology, along with the promising early results of chemotherapeutic treatments for MS have undoubtedly lessened the impact of MS on personal and social functioning. However, work—the role that occupies some one-third of a person's adult life—remains an all too frequent casualty of the physiologic accompaniments of this degenerative disease.

Cognitive Dysfunction

Cognitive deficits associated with the exacerbation and/or progression of MS are arguably the most frustrating aspect of the illness. The rate at which one learns new information, skills, and procedures is often diminished (Franklin et al., 1989), as are short-term memory (Grant et al., 1984), long-term memory (Rao, Leo, & St. Aubin-Faubert, 1989), and abstract reasoning abilities (Halligan et al., 1988). By their own reports, employees with MS identified significant career maintenance barriers resulting from thought-processing and memory deficits in Roessler and Rumrill's (1995a) needs assessment study. Edgley, Sullivan, and Dehoux (1991) showed that the frequency of perceived cognitive problems is directly related to the rate of unemployment among people with MS in Canada. Respondents who indicated that they rarely experienced cognitive problems reported an unemployment rate of 53 percent. Although this is higher than would be expected in the general population, the unemployment rates for people with MS who described the regularity of cognitive problems as *sometimes* (67 percent), *often* (73 percent), and *almost always* (86 percent) were significantly higher. Genevie, Kallos, and Struenig (1987) reported similar findings, noting a significant negative correlation between level of cognitive dysfunction and employment status.

In another investigation, Rao and colleagues (1991) administered neurologic examinations to one hundred people with MS. They used the results of the test battery to classify participants as either "cognitively intact" (n = 52) or "cognitively impaired" (n = 48). Although the two groups did not differ significantly with respect to degree of physical disability or duration of illness, the "intact" group was more likely to be working, engaged in more social and avocational pursuits, and subject to less difficulty with tasks of independent living than the group classified as "impaired."

These findings suggest that cognitive dysfunction has a significant impact on employment status, irrespective of disease-related factors such as physiologic symptoms and duration of illness. Rao, Leo, and St. Aubin-Faubert (1989) recommended further study to improve the timeliness and accuracy of current cognitive deficit assessment instruments. They maintained that this would allow for adaptations in the work setting and enable people with MS to receive formalized cognitive retraining to enhance their employability.

Psychological Factors

The impact of physiologic and cognitive impairments on employment status is partially attributable to the location of CNS lesions, but "the physical aspects of MS do not come close to fully explaining the high rate of unemployment" (LaRocca & Hall, 1990, p. 53). LaRocca and Hall (1990) speculated that the episodic course of MS causes psychological problems which, in turn, lead to diminished employability. These problems include depression, anxiety, euphoria, irritability, and emotional instability (Marsh, Ellison, & Strite, 1983; Minden & Schiffer, 1990).

Emotional Problems

Although multiple sclerosis is often accompanied by emotional and/or psychological problems, people with MS are often not fully aware of the extent of these problems and do not generally equate them with job loss. LaRocca and colleagues (1985) found that only 2.8 percent of unemployed people with MS considered emotional difficulties to be the primary reason for their job loss. Edgley, Sullivan, and Dehoux (1991) also noted that self-reported emotional problems had a much smaller impact on employment status than such factors as gender, age, and physiologic symptoms. Nonetheless, Genevie, Kallos, and Struenig (1987) found that people with MS who identified problems with "affective lability" were significantly less likely to be employed than those who indicated stable emotional patterns.

Job Satisfaction

Job satisfaction has been linked to job tenure and employment status in both the general population (Dawis & Lofquist, 1984) and people with MS (Roessler & Rumrill, 1995a). Roessler and Rumrill (1995a) found that even those with MS who were employed experienced high levels of dissatisfaction with their jobs. Employees with MS (n = 50) were generally dissatisfied with (1) the amount of work they were expected to do (too much); (2) the amount of pay they received (too little); (3) their opportunities for advancement (too few); (4) the training they received on the job (too little); and (5) the recognition afforded them for their work (too little). It should be noted that within the disability community low job satisfaction is not unique to employees with MS. Houser and Chace's (1993) cross-disability study revealed similar levels of dissatisfaction with pay, chance for advancement, and the equity of company policies.

Job Mastery

Roessler and Rumrill (1995a) also described job mastery problems as common psychological impediments to job retention for people with MS. Using an adapted version of Crites's (1990) *Career Mastery Inventory*, they reported frequent job mastery concerns among employees with MS in response to such items as (1) considering what I will do in the future (46 percent); (2) having a plan for where I want to be in my job in the future (40 percent); and (3) believing that others think I do a good job (32

These findings suggest that the medical symptoms of
its unpredictable course make it extremely difficult to
te and act on long-term career plans. It goes without say-
t this uncertainty has a potentially devastating emotional
impact.

Self-Efficacy

In specifying the relationships among the medical symptoms of
MS, its unpredictable course, and its emotional impact, Rumrill
(1993) proposed self-efficacy as the "missing link" between MS
and unemployment. Self-efficacy is defined in Bandura's (1986)
terms to include two domains of expectancy—efficacy expectations and outcome expectations. Efficacy expectations reflect a
person's confidence that he has the skills needed to respond
effectively in a given situation. Outcome expectations refer to the
likelihood that the person will actually attempt a certain task
based on his perception of whether task performance would
result in desirable consequences.

Multiple sclerosis and other severe disabilities have a negative
impact on self-efficacy (Devins & Seland, 1987). It is also well
documented that maintaining a career while coping with a
severe disability such as MS requires the person to take an
active role in overcoming disability-related work limitations
(Gecas, 1989; Gibbs, 1990; Roessler & Rumrill, 1994a, 1994b).
Thus, the relationship between diminished self-efficacy and
unemployment in people with MS can be stated in functional
and theoretical terms: "They (people with MS) do not believe
that they possess the skills required to remove or reduce on-the-
job barriers to their productivity (efficacy expectations), nor do
they have the confidence that such actions will result in desirable outcomes (outcome expectations)" (Roessler & Rumrill,
1994b, p. 55). As a consequence of the influence of self-efficacy, then, many people with MS may leave the workforce prematurely rather than invoke the employment rights to which
they are entitled under Title I of the Americans with Disabilities
Act of 1990 (see Chapter 5).

In concluding their article "Strategies for Enhancing Career
Maintenance Self-Efficacy of People with Multiple Sclerosis,"
Roessler and Rumrill (1994b) recommended "early interventions"

to assist employees with MS in (1) identifying on-the-job barriers to productivity; (2) understanding their rights to reasonable accommodations; and (3) developing techniques for communicating their needs to their employers. Chapters 3 and 4 of this text provide detailed descriptions of how these and other employment-enhancement strategies have been implemented at sites across the country.

Workplace Variables

Most contemporary theories of psychology consider human behavior to be the product of reciprocation between personal and environmental factors (see Chapter 3). This discussion has so far focused on the intrapersonal aspects of MS that impinge on employment prospects. A few researchers have examined the work environment for contributors to the sharp decline in employment that awaits many people with MS soon after diagnosis.

Work Performance

Gulick, Yam, and Touw (1989) viewed the person-environment interaction as an essential consideration in evaluating work performance of people with MS. Their qualitative study revealed that physical limitations, MS-related symptoms, and environmental factors were reciprocally related to job performance and, consequently, to job retention. They emphasized the need to empower employees with MS to "collect data as a basis for judging their own functional level and self-care demands related to their work performance" (Gulick, Yam, & Touw, 1989, p. 309).

Taking an encompassing view of work, which included employment, activities of daily living, and coping with symptoms, Gulick (1992) attributed diminished work performance to *work impediments* such as mobility problems, fine motor difficulties, deterioration of general body state, cognitive dysfunction, pain, and environmental barriers. She suggested that people with MS could improve their work performance via such *work enhancers* as job adjustments, environmental adjustments and assistive technology, social support, and healthful self-care practices.

Career Adjustment Barriers: Worksite Accessibility and Essential Functions

The Minnesota Theory of Work Adjustment (Dawis & Lofquist, 1984) holds that job tenure (longevity) is a function of satisfaction and satisfactoriness. Satisfaction refers to the extent to which a job provides sufficient internal and external reinforcement for the individual, whereas satisfactoriness reflects how well the person performs the job. Crites (1976) proposed job tenure (satisfaction + satisfactoriness) to be largely determined by one's ability to overcome thwarting conditions, or barriers, at work.

Conceptualizing the medical and psychological effects of MS as internal barriers to career adjustment, Roessler and Rumrill (1995a) examined perceived worksite barriers for their relationship to feelings of job satisfaction and job mastery (satisfactoriness) among a sample of fifty employees with MS in Indiana and Kentucky. Using the Work Experience Survey (WES) (Roessler, 1995; see Chapter 3), they found that the number of disability-related barriers to worksite accessibility and performance of essential functions of the job correlated significantly and positively with the number of satisfaction and mastery problems reported. As a result, they developed a simple prediction equation to assess what they termed "at risk" status: the more accessibility and essential function barriers one perceives on the job, the lower the levels of job satisfaction and mastery and, thus, the greater the risk of job loss.

The specific on-the-job barriers that placed participants in Roessler and Rumrill's (1995a) study "at risk" of losing their jobs represented a range as broad and varied as the medical symptoms of MS. In the area of worksite accessibility, respondents reported an average of twenty-eight barriers. Because hypersensitivity to heat is one of the most common physiologic effects of MS, it is not surprising that the temperature of the workplace was the most frequently mentioned barrier, identified by 47 percent of participants. Other commonly noted accessibility obstacles were hazards (27 percent), entrances (22 percent), and stairs and steps (22 percent).

With regard to performance of essential functions, respondents identified an average of nearly twelve barriers that had the potential to threaten job retention. Participants reported significant problems with job demands that required physical abilities such as handling (45 percent), seeing well (34 percent), considerable walking (30 percent), working eight hours (28 percent), standing part of the time (28 percent), standing all day (24 percent), and use of the lower extremities (24 percent). Essential function barriers related to cognitive abilities included thought processing (44 percent), immediate memory (40 percent), short-term memory (38 percent), and long-term memory (26 percent). Task-related abilities presented frequent problems in the areas of writing (48 percent), remembering (48 percent), speaking/communicating (46 percent), working under stress or deadlines (42 percent), repetitive work (24 percent), and work pace (24 percent).

Advocating for proactive responses from rehabilitation professionals to assist people with MS in maintaining employment, Roessler and Rumrill (1995a, p. 12) interpreted their findings as follows:

> Early interventions to remove barriers to access and performance would increase the likelihood that employees with MS would retain their jobs because barrier removal influences two important predictors of job retention—job satisfaction and job satisfactoriness. Interventions are also needed to lessen the dissatisfaction that people with MS have with specific aspects of their work such as work load, amount of pay, advancement, and on-the-job training.

Employer Attitudes and Reactions of Coworkers

Another worksite variable that influences the likelihood that a person with MS will retain employment is the reaction of the employer and coworkers to disability–related needs. Employer reactions to MS are not always negative. In a study in New Zealand, more than 90 percent of those with MS who had disclosed their illness to employers regarded employer reactions as "somewhat sympathetic" or "very sympathetic." Sympathy may not be the most desirable response to a disclosure of MS, but employee-employer understanding is essential to the job retention process.

In Belgium, Ketelaer and colleagues (1993) found that employer attitudes and interactions with coworkers influenced the willingness of employees to request MS-related "adaptations" at work. Rumrill, Roessler, and Denny (in press) linked the act of requesting on-the-job accommodations to self-efficacy, which has been associated with MS and employment status in several investigations (Devins & Seland, 1987; Gecas, 1989; Roessler & Rumrill, 1994b; Rumrill, 1993). Thus, integrating these findings forges a direct connection between environmental and personal factors related to the employment of people with MS: reactions of employers and coworkers influence the employee's willingness to ask for needed help on the job; willingness to ask for help influences self-efficacy, and vice versa; and the reciprocal relationship between self-efficacy and willingness to ask for help influences the person's prospects for continued employment.

Job Type and Working Conditions

In 1985, LaRocca and colleagues asserted that, although occupational type was related to an individual's overall psychosocial adjustment to MS, it was unrelated to employment status. Such factors as disability level, age, gender, and educational attainment were much stronger predictors of job retention and loss within the American MS community. More recently, however, Ketelaer and colleagues (1993) reported that people employed in the medical field and in jobs that required them to work out-of-doors, stand for long periods of time, and exert physical strength were significantly more likely to lose their jobs than those working under other occupational conditions. They also found higher rates of unemployment among people who could not travel independently and among those who had not been members of labor unions.

Rozin and colleagues (1975) reported that Israelis with MS who worked in jobs that required a four-year college degree were more likely to maintain employment than less educated workers. They also found higher rates of employment among people whose career fields required little physical exertion.

Availability of On-the-Job Accommodations

In another study, Duggan, Fagan, and Yateman (1993) simply asked unemployed people with MS why they had left their jobs. Approximately 75 percent reported that they stopped working voluntarily, and worksite barriers were frequently noted as a reason for that choice. These on-the-job obstacles included less-than-helpful employee assistance programs (which were viewed as being exclusively concerned with alcoholism and other drug abuse) and poor access to reasonable accommodations. Only one in five respondents had received accommodations in the workplace, and many believed that they could have benefited from such arrangements as home-based work, educating employers about MS, and individual employment counseling. They also felt that information concerning the Americans with Disabilities Act, legal rights, health insurance, and Social Security Disability Insurance would have helped them to retain employment. Significantly, respondents seldom attributed their unemployment to issues of disclosure, absenteeism, safety, or interpersonal relationships. It should also be noted that many unemployed people with MS leave the workforce for non MS-related reasons. LaRocca and colleagues (1985) found that 37.1 percent of non-working people with MS had left their jobs due to pregnancy, marriage, relocation, or retirement. Rozin and colleagues (1975) found that 72 percent of respondents viewed their MS as having no impact whatsoever on employment; only 18 percent reported losing their jobs as a result of the illness, and 10 percent had changed careers as a result of acquiring MS.

The importance of reasonable accommodations to employees with MS was upheld in Roessler and Rumrill's (1995a) findings. Although participants in their study ($n = 50$) reported many and appreciable worksite barriers, they also reported using a number of on-the-job accommodations (56) to address those problems. In order of frequency, these involved installation of new equipment (17), restructuring of the job (11), modification of work schedules (9), restructuring of existing facilities (8), change in location of the worksite (5), reassignment to another position (3), provision of personal assistance (2), and modification of equipment (1).

In general, job retention interventions for people with disabilities are most effective when priority is placed on helping the person to continue in his or her present position (Matkin, 1995). The same appears to be true for those with MS, and reasonable accommodations at the worksite constitute a central theme of contemporary MS research on career maintenance (Rumrill, 1993; Rumrill, Roessler, & Denny, in press; Sumner, 1995). Within a subsample of successfully employed workers with MS, Kraft, Freal, and Coryell (1986) noted that the vast majority were employed in the jobs they had held at the time of diagnosis, and that very few had changed jobs since the onset of their illness. These findings indicate that rehabilitation services should be introduced immediately after diagnosis to assist individuals in keeping their jobs. In that effort, accommodation planning must be specific to the person's present work environment and job demands.

Given the range and severity of physiologic, cognitive, and psychological symptoms, it is not surprising that people with MS have encountered numerous and imposing barriers at the worksite. Experts have drawn connections between illness-related factors and work performance, physical accessibility of the workplace, essential function barriers, employer discrimination and co-worker responses, and the availability of on-the-job accommodations. Several of the intervention strategies outlined in Chapter 4 address the issue of worksite barrier removal, but more research is needed concerning proactive strategies to enable people with MS to continue working as their illness progresses.

Work Disincentives in the Social Security Program

LaRocca's (1995) estimate that only one-third of unemployed Americans with MS are interested in rejoining the labor force is in part attributable to financial disincentives in the Social Security Disability Insurance (SSDI) and Supplemental Security Income (SSI) programs. In 1987, for example, 39,100 people with MS received SSDI benefits at an annual cost of more than $20 million (LaRocca, 1995). Minden (1995) calculated a lifetime cost of $495,845 (1991 dollars) per SSDI recipient. The total cost of maintaining people with MS on SSDI rolls has undoubtedly increased in recent years as a result of such factors as (1) general inflation, (2) escalating health care costs, and (3) increased prevalence of the illness.

The fact that SSDI cash and income transfer benefits are intended only for those who have withdrawn from the labor force creates an inherent impediment to any vocational rehabilitation initiative. Efforts to help people with disabilities return to the labor market are seriously undermined by the very real threat that they are likely to have their benefits discontinued if rehabilitation services result in job placements (Rubin & Roessler, 1995).

For people with MS, the stable, guaranteed stream of income offered by SSDI is often preferable to the much less stable prospect of holding a job while coping with a chronic progressive disease. A 1987 survey of 439 members of the New York City Chapter of the National Multiple Sclerosis Society found the receipt of SSDI benefits to be a significant inhibitor of respondents' intentions to re-enter the workforce (Genevie, Kallos, & Struenig, 1987). Moreover, readers who have enrolled in SSDI or any other social security program know how arduous and lengthy the application and eligibility determination process can be. Hence, the possibility, even probability, of a work-handicapping exacerbation of the illness makes the person with MS even less likely to risk discontinuation of benefits; there is no assurance that SSDI enrollment could be quickly reinstated if she becomes unable to continue working, and an extended period without benefits may result.

Health Insurance Issues

Many people with MS who leave their jobs enter the SSDI program. In most cases, the monthly stipend of SSDI is accompanied by government health insurance through the Medicare program. Although it is far from perfect, Medicare offers guaranteed coverage *with no preexisting condition exclusions* for qualified recipients. Hence, the individual is not subject to annual or lifetime "caps," nor is he at risk of having coverage denied or discontinued because of the actuarially computed cost of his condition (Mahoney, 1995).

Keniston (1995) noted that Medicare serves as a desirable alternative to private insurance for many Americans with multiple sclerosis. He further suggested that one of the primary factors associated with the decision not to work is the fear of losing government health care benefits and placing responsibility for insurance coverage in the hands of private carriers.

The Catch-22 obstacle to employment for millions of Americans is the fact that a chronic illness such as MS both creates a greater need for health insurance coverage than ever before and makes it increasingly difficult for those diagnosed to receive and/or maintain said coverage. Therefore, it is troubling but not surprising that so many qualified and productive people have elected to prematurely disengage from the labor force. LaRocca and Hall (1990) demonstrated that extending the three-year Medicare continuation policy in the SSDI program (to thirteen years) had dramatic results; approximately two-thirds of those with MS who completed *Operation Job Match: MS Back to Work* were still employed as of this writing, more than ten years after the inception of the program. However, the Social Security Administration remains interminably slow to adopt broad-based reforms that would truly encourage people with disabilities to seek, secure, and maintain competitive employment.

Summary

Determining the correlates of unemployment among individuals with MS is complicated by the variety and scope of symptoms related to the illness, which make it necessary for investigators to consider a number of interactive factors in explaining why so many people with MS leave the workforce prematurely.

Demographic characteristics such as gender, socioeconomic status, and age are related to unemployment in people with MS. Specifically, women, older workers, and those with higher family incomes are most likely to leave the workforce after diagnosis. Significantly, most people with MS who stop working do so voluntarily. Additional research is needed concerning relationships among race, geography, and unemployment.

As might be expected, the physiologic symptoms of MS explain some of the variance in employment status. Physical limitations (especially mobility problems) and fatigue are commonly cited reasons for job loss. To a lesser extent, visual impairment, loss of coordination, and incontinence have also been attributed. Additionally, disease-related variables such as age at onset, duration of illness, and the progression of symptoms have been shown to predict whether one continues working.

Cognitive and other psychological problems have a significant impact on employment. Memory problems, thought processing difficulties, emotional instability, job satisfaction and mastery concerns, and low self-efficacy have all been linked to poor prospects for job retention by people with MS.

At the workplace itself, many on-the-job variables have been examined for their contributions to the career maintenance difficulties experienced by people with MS. These include the performance of essential functions, worksite accessibility, employer attitudes and coworker reactions, and the availability of reasonable accommodations.

Last but not least are disincentives in the SSDI program. The stability of social security payments in comparison to competitive employment is a work-inhibiting factor for people with MS, as is the prospect of having Medicare insurance benefits discontinued and subjecting oneself to the seemingly whimsical private-pay insurance industry.

In his synthesis report to the National Multiple Sclerosis Society on employment and MS, LaRocca (1995, pp. 5–6) proposed that researchers and service providers consider the following strategies in addressing predictors of unemployment such as those presented in this chapter:

1. We need to focus our efforts more broadly on quality of life including meaningful substitutes to employment. . . . People (with MS) need help to plan realistically without giving up.

2. Job-retention programs need to address more than just employment issues. . . .

3. Empowerment models, in which people with MS assume the major responsibility for their own fates, need to be utilized more extensively.

4. More education programs are needed to inform people with MS about such matters as their legal rights, job accommodations, medical and psychological issues, health insurance, and SSDI work incentives.

5. More liaison is needed with employers to help them learn about other matters, such as the special needs of people with MS, the nature of job accommodations, absenteeism, and employer tax incentives for hiring people with disabilities.

6. A proactive approach is needed to maximize utilization of the Americans with Disabilities Act, Social Security Disability work incentives, and other legislation since people with MS seem to underutilize these opportunities.

7. Longitudinal research is needed to understand why some remain
working while others do not.

These and other research and service priorities are addressed in
greater detail in subsequent chapters.

Chapter 3

Vocational Assessment Strategies

Richard T. Roessler

Editor's Note: *The following chapter addresses strategies for assessing the medical, psychological, and social aspects of career development for people with multiple sclerosis. It is intended primarily for health care professionals, social workers, psychologists, and rehabilitation practitioners who have a basic working knowledge of psychometric principles. For the benefit of readers who do not have a background in measurement, technical terms are defined in the text.*

One theme recurs throughout this book: multiple sclerosis (MS) is a severe mid-career disability that presents significant challenges to adults who are determined to resume or retain employment. Indicative of the complications associated with the disease, the unemployment rate for people with MS equals or exceeds that reported by the general population of adults with disabilities (Rao et al., 1991). For the most part, barriers to the retention of employment result from the gravity, pervasiveness, and unpredictability of the symptoms themselves (Falvo, 1991). At the same time, these symptoms tend to have a cumulative psychological effect that results in uncertainty about one's life and future. That uncertainty, in turn, serves to magnify the impact of individual physical and cognitive symptoms associated with the disease process (LaRocca et al., 1985). This chapter describes assessment strategies that help to clarify the way that MS both impairs functioning in career roles and produces psychological uncertainty about the future. As Goldberg (1992) pointed out, the probability that a person will return to work depends in large part on the impact of disability on work-related skills, motivation to work, and optimism about the future.

Department of Rehabilitation, University of Arkansas

Assessments recommended for people with MS provide insights into the personal preferences, functional limitations, rehabilitation outlook, and perceived barriers that affect success in coping with the effects of physical and psychological symptoms of the illness. The reader is reminded, however, of one of the basic premises of psychological assessment supported by Goldberg's (1992) research: in the case of people with adventitious disabilities such as MS, the best predictors of future interests, values, and vocational plans are the person's past interests, values, and vocational accomplishments. Indeed, for acquired disabling conditions, prior commitments and preferences have more influence on the person's vocational choice than does the severity of the disability (Goldberg, 1992). Hence, rehabilitation professionals should concentrate first on helping the person maintain continuity in his vocational life by retaining employment held before the onset of disability, turning to other vocational assessments and placement strategies when necessary to identify transferable skills and potential jobs with compatible skill demands.

A Philosophy of Assessment

Because of their impact on individual functioning in a variety of areas (mobility, strength, cognition, and vision), the symptoms of multiple sclerosis are disruptive to the person's career in the broadest sense of the term *career*. For example, the more encompassing career development theories define career as including adult roles such as employee, citizen, learner, family member, and participant in leisure activities (McDaniel & Gysbers, 1992). Hence, although this chapter focuses on issues of vocational evaluation, it does not intend to imply that the effect of MS on other daily living and community roles is unimportant. The interdependence of career roles is stressed, requiring that the rehabilitation professional explore how MS affects multiple career roles and how limitations in performance of these roles impinge on the person's capability to seek, acquire, and retain employment.

In addition to the career emphasis, the philosophy of assessment underlying this chapter includes a person-in-environment perspective that integrates the traditional trait and factor approach with the ecological approach. The trait and factor paradigm is retained because it defines person variables that are fairly stable even in the face of a significant disability such as MS. Such attributes of the person as vocational interests, aptitudes, skills, self-concept, and preferences for work climates and reinforcers fall into the trait/factor category (Hershenson, 1992, 1987; Kosciulek, 1993).

The ecological perspective is also useful because it stresses that environmental variables are equally important for understanding the vocational outcomes of a person with a disability. As Dobren (1994) noted, these ecological variables include the attitudes of others (e.g., reactions of family and employer to the disability and resumption of employment) and the presses in the environment (e.g., the nature of the tasks or expectations that define the career setting in which the person is expected to function). Dobren (1994) also described how severe disabilities such as MS alter the context in which the person functions by creating new variables with which the person has little or no experience, such as architectural barriers, attitudes of physicians and other health care providers, and financial disincentives posed by disability benefit programs. Therefore, the assessor must have a perspective that encompasses the person, the context, and the interaction of the two. One must understand the tasks and expectations of the job that a person holds (environment) to know which disability-related limitations (person) create significant barriers to performance of essential job functions. Because the effects of MS vary so widely among individuals, on-the-job barriers must be considered on the basis of each person's specific job duties. For example, a high school mathematics teacher coping with mobility restrictions as a result of MS is less vocationally handicapped than a farmer or construction worker dealing with the same or even less severe mobility impairments.

As noted, focusing assessment on physical limitations alone without examining the demands of a specific career role can provide only a partial understanding of the person's needs. Knowledge of both allows the professional to intervene with both the individual's capacities and the demands of the environment. Thus, coupling the trait and factor perspective with the ecological outlook provides a more encompassing view of assessment and its implications. With the dual (person/environment) point of view, the professional understands that interventions are not directed solely at changing the person. They also must affect the situation in which the person functions, with the end result being congruence between the job demands and the person's capabilities as mediated by accommodative strategies that include job restructuring, technology utilization, and flexible scheduling. The remainder of this chapter provides an overview of assessment strategies and measures that, when viewed in their entirety, are sensitive to the person and the demands of the setting. Results from such instruments provide practical information on the person's needs for skill-building experiences, technology utilization, and environmental modifications.

Capitalizing on Continuity

Given the research-based conclusion that the best predictors of future vocational preferences are past vocational preferences, the rehabilitation professional working with people with MS should first involve the person in examining the feasibility of returning to the same job with the same employer as quickly as possible (Matkin, 1995). If such employment is possible, the next step involves identifying barriers at the workplace that impede vocational success and identifying reasonable accommodations that will reduce or remove those barriers. An assessment strategy for identifying workplace barriers, the Work Experience Survey (WES), is described later in the chapter.

If the person cannot return to the same job/same employer, the rehabilitation professional can assist him in completing a vocational analysis, with the end goal being identification of similar or related employment roles available in the local community. Described in recent rehabilitation resources (Roessler & Rubin, 1992; Rubin & Roessler, 1995), the vocational analysis may be no more involved than reviewing existing occupational information resources such as the *Dictionary of Occupational Titles* (1991) and the annual *Occupational Outlook Handbook* produced by the United States Department of Labor in order to identify feasible job options and develop a job-seeking plan.

The *Dictionary of Occupational Titles (DOT)* is useful because it enables a person to identify additional job titles in the same industry and occupational classification in which she previously worked. Divided into nine industry categories, the *DOT* presents information on over 20,000 jobs. Given the occupational title in the *DOT* for the person's previous job, it is possible to determine its job family and related occupational titles. These related titles provide valuable vocational possibilities that the person might consider pursuing. For example, knowing that the person worked as a shipping and receiving clerk, coded in the *DOT* as 222.387–050, one can locate other related jobs in the 200 category that might be of interest, such as inventory clerk (222.387–026).

Jobs of interest located in the *DOT* are described in detail, including information on job duties and related occupations. For more up-to-date information on the occupation, the *Occupational Outlook Handbook* published by the Department of Labor is a useful resource (U.S. Department of Labor, annual). Current information is provided on the educational and training requirements for the position, the occupational outlook for the job, and the salary/wage range typically associated with the position.

Based on information on the physical demands and job duties of positions described in resources such as the *DOT*, the rehabilitation professional can help evaluate the feasibility of vocational alternatives by assessing the person/job congruence (Parker, Szymanski, & Hanley-Maxwell, 1989). Parker, Szymanski, and Hanley-Maxwell (1989) listed the person and job variables that must be considered in establishing this person/job match. Using intake interview information and existing evaluation data, the rehabilitation professional can create a synthesis of the person's medical and educational history, past vocational training, work history, current situation, and current work-related strengths and limitations. This case history is extremely important because research with people who have multiple sclerosis indicates that elements of a person's history are related to employment outcomes. Poor employment outcomes are associated with (1) the chronic progression of MS; (2) greater physical involvement including spasticity, lack of coordination, and disturbances in bowel and bladder function; and (3) being female and older (Kornblith, LaRocca, & Baum, 1986). Larsen (1990) reported that adjustment scores in the vocational domain for people with MS were higher for those who had employment histories or had attended college.

As a result of the vocational analysis, the person has a list of feasible vocational alternatives that should be evaluated for (1) compatibility with her skills and interests, and (2) availability in the local community. Recommending a job analysis to estimate person/job compatibility, Parker, Szymanski, and Hanley-Maxwell (1989) stressed the need for general information about the employer and specific information about the job. The size and stability of the company, availability of employer-provided transportation for employees, and the employer's history of support for and retention of people with disabilities are examples of general employer information. Gathered through job analyses, job-specific data include the tasks required in the position, the speed of production involved, quality and quantity standards, and equipment used in the position.

The most promising job titles identified in the vocational analysis provide the foundation for beginning a traditional job search strategy including such steps as building one's job lead network, accessing information on current job openings, organizing the job search, and recording the results of job-seeking contacts. LaRocca and Hall (1990) described the use of job-seeking groups in their MS Job-Raising program (see Chapter 4), which included didactic instruction in job-seeking and networking as well as personal support among people with MS.

Other strategies exist for initiating the vocational analysis process that capitalize on continuity, i.e., the desirability of helping the person with MS resume employment similar to that held before the onset or exacerbation of symptoms. One technique requires knowledge of the work reinforcers (those factors that encourage a person to continue working) available in a job and the titles of other jobs providing similar types of reinforcers. In the Minnesota Theory of Work Adjustment (Dawis, 1987), twenty discrete work reinforcers are defined, such as ability utilization, creativity, compensation, authority, and activity. Each job has a characteristic pattern of reinforcers, and each person has a characteristic set of preferences for these reinforcers. To increase the probability of job satisfaction, the person with MS must identify new job titles that are available in the local community and provide access to (1) his preferred reinforcers, and (2) job duties compatible with existing skills and physical capacities.

Although estimates of reinforcer preferences on the part of the person and reinforcer availability on the part of the job may be generated from interviews with the person and her supervisors and coworkers, a written assessment measure that the person with MS can complete is also available. The Minnesota

Importance Questionnaire (MIQ) enables respondents to indicate their personal preferences among the twenty work reinforcers. The resulting needs profile of the person is related to information on the work reinforcers characteristic of a wide range of jobs, and a list of job/person matches is produced as an outcome of the computer scoring process for the MIQ. This list of job titles includes positions that the person would find satisfying based on the need/reinforcer match principle (Dawis & Lofquist, 1984). The next step is to identify compatible positions available in the local community and to assist the person in organizing a job search plan targeted to those jobs and employers.

Research with the Minnesota Theory of Work Adjustment has demonstrated that satisfaction with one's work is only one of the factors that affects tenure on the job. The other important factor is satisfactoriness on the job, i.e., the ability to perform the job as evaluated by one's supervisor or employer. Consistent with the ecological perspective advocated earlier, satisfactoriness is a function of the person's being able to perform job-specific tasks in a manner that meets the employer's quantity and quality standards. Although the potential for job satisfactoriness should be analyzed in detail prior to placement, it is also possible to assess on-the-job satisfactoriness using the Minnesota Satisfactoriness Scales (MSS) (Dawis & Lofquist, 1984). Completed by the supervisor or employer, the MSS contains items addressing the person's work capacities, comparability with other workers in the position, and suitability for a pay raise and promotion. If gathered early enough in the worker's adjustment to the new position, MSS data can highlight areas in which the person needs additional support, training, or accommodations to cope more effectively with the demands of the new position. If made as soon as possible, such post-placement adjustments increase the probability of satisfactoriness, which, when coupled with satisfaction, is predictive of long-term tenure on the job.

Career Role Performance

In keeping with the career theme and the ecological perspective described earlier, Gulick (1991, 1992) presented several assessments useful with people who have MS. Defining work as any activity that requires the expenditure of energy to maintain the person's existence, self-esteem, or remuneration, she developed the Work Assessment Scale (WAS), which enables people with MS to describe the factors that impede their capacity to do work (WAS-I) and the factors that have the potential to reduce or remove those impediments (work enhancers, WAS-E).

By completing the WAS, people who have multiple sclerosis can describe how the following factors impede their ability to complete work (WAS-I): impairments in mobility, hand functioning, cognitive functioning, and general body state; and the existence of pain, environmental barriers, or jobs that require heavy labor. The seven factors of the work impediment scale had theta reliability coefficients (a measure of consistency among items within a particular factor or scale) ranging from .73 to .90 and demonstrated expectable concurrent validity relationships with subscales from measures of daily living skills and symptoms of MS (Gulick, 1991).

Valuable for suggesting interventions to increase people's capacities to function in career roles, information from the WAS-E scale helps to determine whether changes are needed in areas such as environmental or job modifications, level of social support, beneficial health practices, and personal attributes and strengths. Internal consistency of the WAS-E subscales was acceptable, with theta coefficients ranging from .66 (Healthful Practices) to .81 (Personal Attributes). Over a two- to three-week period, test-retest correlation coefficients ranged from .68 to .82. Again, evidence of concurrent validity for the WAS-E occurred in certain expectable relationships between WAS-E subscales and subscales of a daily living scale for people with MS (Gulick, 1991). Abstracted from the WAS-E, a sampling of conditions or activities that are considered work enhancing is provided in Table 3-1.

As Gulick (1991) noted, the WAS has a number of possible applications in the assessment of people with MS. When used in combination by health and rehabilitation professionals, the WAS-I and WAS-E result in identification not only of work impediments but also of strategies to reduce or remove those impediments. The identification of barriers alone (WAS-I) is obviously only a first step toward helping people with MS perform more effectively in areas such as personal care, homemaking, and employment (WAS-E). With information from the WAS-E, it is also possible to recommend a multifaceted approach to barrier removal

Table 3-1. Work Adjustment Scale-E

Sample Enhancing Conditions and Activities[a]

Job Adjustment
  Sit down job
  Plan tasks when energy is highest

Environmental Adjustment/Adaptive Devices
  Adaptive equipment/devices
  Conveniently arranged supplies

Support
  Emotional support
  Assistance with tasks

Personal Attributes
  Positive attitude
  Control of stress

Personal Health Habits
  Good night's sleep
  Peaceful atmosphere

[a]Selected from Work Enhancement Scale-E (Gulick, 1991)

that may require changes (1) in the person's interpretation of the situation; (2) in the person's health practices with regard to diet, rest, and surroundings; and/or (3) in the nature of the situational demands that the person must satisfy.

Gulick reported on two other scales of interest in the assessment of MS and its implications for the individual. The fifteen-item ADL Self-Care Scale (ADL-MS) includes four areas of daily functioning that affect the person's performance in a variety of career roles (Gulick, 1987, 1991; Gulick & Bugg, 1992). The four ADL areas included in the scale are fine and gross motor (eating, dressing, bathing, transfer, walking, and travel), socializing/recreation (activities inside and outside the home), sensory/communication (reading, writing, telephoning), and intimacy (confiding, expressions of love, sexual activity). Scores on the ADL-MS correlated as expected with scales on the WAS (Gulick, 1991).

The MS-Related Symptoms Checklist (MS-RS) is another valuable instrument (Gulick, 1991; Gulick & Bugg, 1992). By the term *instrument*, psychologists mean the form or device used to measure a particular construct. If assessors wish to gain more detailed information regarding the symptoms that people with MS are experiencing, they can administer the MS-RS. Covering a variety of symptoms (twenty-six in all), the MS-RS consists of five factors (symptom clusters) that include twenty-two of the twenty-six symptoms measured. The five symptom clusters are termed *motor, brainstem, sensory, mental-emotions,* and *elimination,* with the number of items in each factor ranging from three to five (see Table 3-2). As was the case with the ADL-MS, scores on the MS-RS correlated as expected with the WAS. Additionally, scores on both measures revealed significant negative changes over a five-year time period for people with MS, particularly for people who had been diagnosed more recently (Gulick & Bugg, 1992).

Table 3-2.   MS-Related Symptom Scale (MS-RS) Symptom Clusters[a]

Motor
   Arm and leg weakness
   Spasms
   Tremors
   Knee locking
   Balance problems
   Falling

Brainstem
   Double and blurred vision
   Difficulty swallowing
   Forgetfulness

Sensory
   Pain
   Burning
   Numbness
   Pins and needles

[a]*Mental-Emotions*
   Loneliness
   Depression
   Anxiety

Elimination
   Urine frequency: day and night
   Trouble making toilet: day and night

[a] From Gulick & Bugg, 1992

Work Role Performance

Hershenson (1990) described the initial impact of disability as affecting the work competencies of the individual. The negative impact of an adventitious disability such as multiple sclerosis on work competencies radiates to other aspects of the person such as self-image and work goals. Hence, instruments are needed to determine how a disability affects the work-related competencies of the person and other directly relevant variables such as job mastery and job satisfaction, all of which have a bearing on work role performance. Gulick's (1991) Work Assessment Scale (WAS) is useful in this regard, as is the Work Experience Survey, another measure that combines the trait/factor and ecological assessment orientations of this chapter.

The Work Experience Survey

The Work Experience Survey (WES) (Roessler, 1995) is a structured interview that enables rehabilitation professionals to determine where MS has created work-related barriers. These barriers may limit the person's capacity to gain access to the worksite, perform essential functions, and/or maintain job mastery and satisfaction.

In completing the WES interview with a rehabilitation professional, the person with MS identifies not only barriers to productivity but also the accommodations needed to reduce or remove those barriers. With information from the WES, the individual is in a position to direct his or her own accommodation planning consistent with employment provisions and protections in Title I of the ADA (see Chapter 5). Administered in a face-to-face or telephone interview by a rehabilitation professional, the WES consists of six sections: (1) background information on the respondent, (2) an accessibility checklist, (3) an essential job functions checklist, (4) a job mastery survey, (5) a job satisfaction survey, and (6) an accommodation plan.

The accommodation plan describes how techniques such as job restructuring, worksite modification, and/or the addition of new technology would enable the person to maintain productivity on the job. Information from the sections of the WES, described in the paragraphs to follow, is necessary if the rehabilitation professional is to prepare a thorough case study describing the factors that positively and negatively affect job retention for the person with MS (Roessler & Gottcent, 1994; Roessler & Rumrill, 1995a, 1995c).

Assessing Accessibility

Adapted from a checklist published by the President's Committee on Employment of People with Disabilities (1985), the accessibility section addresses barriers that the worker may experience in entering the worksite, using necessary services and facilities, and exiting the worksite in emergency situations (see Table 3-3). If an accessibility issue is not in the checklist, a space is provided for the respondent to list additional accessibility problems. The final question asks the person to describe solutions for his or her two most important accessibility barriers.

Assessing Essential Job Functions

Adapted from the RehabMatch program, Department of Labor research (Greenwood, Johnson, Wilson, & Schriner, 1988), and recommendations from employment specialists familiar with MS and other severe disabilities, the section on essential job functions is divided into six categories: physical abilities, cognitive abilities, task-related abilities, social abilities, working conditions, and company policies (see Table 3–4). This section enables the person to check any essential job functions or work conditions that constitute problems. The final question in the section asks the individual to describe two potentially helpful accommodations. These accommodations might involve one or more of the strategies suggested in Title I of the Americans with Disabilities Act (ADA), such as restructuring of existing facilities, restructuring of the job, modification of work schedules, reassignment to other positions, modification of equipment, installation of new equipment, flexible personal leave policies, provision of qualified readers or interpreters, and modification of application and examination pro-

Table 3-3. Assessing Accessibility

Section II. Accessibility: Check (4) any problems you have getting to, from, or around on your job. List any other accessibility problems not included in the list. Describe solutions for your two most important accessibility barriers.

___Parking	___Bathrooms	___Temperature
___Public walks	___Water fountains	___Ventilation
___Passenger loading zones	___Public telephone	___Hazards
___Entrance	___Elevators	___Identification signs/labels
___Stairs/Steps	___Lighting	___Access to personnel offices
___Floors/Floor covering	___Warning devices	___Access to general use areas
___Seating/Tables	___Evacuation routes	

List any other accessibility problems:

#1 _____

_____

#2 _____

_____

Describe solutions for your two most important accessibility barriers.

#1 _____

_____

#2 _____

_____

Table 3-4. Assessing Essential Functions

Section III. Essential job functions: Check (4) any essential job functions or conditions* that pose problems for you. Describe the two most important job modifications that you need, e.g., modifying existing equipment, adding new technology, or changing the type of work you do.

Physical Abilities
- ✓ Working 8 hours
- ___Standing all day
- ___Standing part of the time
- ___Working with others
- ___Walking for 8 hours

- ___Some kneeling
- ___Some stooping

- ___Some climbing
- ___Much pulling
- ___Much pushing
- ___Much talking
- ___Seeing well
- ___Hearing well
- ___Handling
- ___Raising arms above shoulders
- ___Using both hands
- ___Using both legs
- ___Using left hand
- ___Using right hand
- ___Using left leg
- ___Using right leg
- ___Lifting over 100 lbs.
- ___Lifting 51–100 lbs.
- ___Lifting 26–50 lbs.
- ___Lifting 11–25 lbs.

- ___Lifting 0–10 lbs.
- ___Prolonged sitting

Cognitive Abilities
- ___Immediate memory
- ___Short-term memory

- ___Judgment: safety

- ___Judgment: interpersonal
- ___Thought processing

- ___Reasoning
- ___Problem solving
- ___Planning
- ___Organizing

Task Related Abilities
- ___Repetitive work
- ✓ Work pace/sequencing
- ✓ Variety of duties
- ✓ Perform under stress/ deadlines
- ___Little feedback on performance
- ___Read written instructions
- ___Able and licensed to drive
- ___Attain precise standards/limits
- ___Follow specific instructions
- ___Writing
- ___Remembering
- ___Speaking/Communicating

- ✓ Initiating work activities
- ___Use telephone

Social Abilities
- ___Working alone
- ___Working around others
- ___Long-term memory

- ___Interacting with supervisors
- ___Supervising others
- ___Working with hostile others

Working Conditions
- ___Too hot
- ___Too cold
- ___Temperature changes
- ___Too wet
- ___Too humid
- ___Slippery surfaces
- ___Obstacles in path
- ___Dust
- ___Fumes
- ___Odors
- ___Noise
- ___Outdoors
- ___Sometimes outdoors
- ___Always inside

Company Policies
- ✓ Inflexible work schedules
- ___No accrual of sick leave
- ✓ Lack of flextime
- ✓ No "comp" time
- ___Inflexible job descriptions
- ✓ Vague job descriptions
- ___Infrequent reviews of job descriptions
- ___Rigid sick/vacation leave policies

Describe the two job modifications that would be most helpful to you, e.g., restructuring of the job, modification of work schedules, reassignment to another position, modification of equipment, or provision of readers and interpreters.

#1_____

_____

#2_____

_____

*Adapted from *RehabMatch*. Arkansas Research and Training Center in Vocational Rehabilitation.

cedures. For example, problems encountered in performing essential functions involving cognitive operations (e.g., memory) could be resolved if the person dictated notes from meetings using a hand-held recorder. Mobility limitations become less problematic if the person's desk computer is linked to an electronic mail system. Finally, a flexible work schedule that allows the person to rest during the work day and work later in the evening is an effective response to the fatigue associated with MS.

Assessing Job Mastery

The job mastery scale (Coefficient Alpha = .74) (Roessler & Rumrill, 1995a) was adapted from *The Career Mastery Inventory* (CMI) developed by John Crites (1990). In addition to providing his permission for use of the items, Crites determined that the content of the items was appropriate for assessing job mastery concerns. The abbreviated measure includes items representing the six domains of *The Career Mastery Inventory*: getting the job done, fitting into the workforce, learning the ropes, getting along with others, getting ahead, and planning the next career step. At the close of the section, the respondent is asked to describe one solution for each of his two top priority job mastery concerns (see Table 3-5).

Assessing Job Satisfaction

Presented in Table 3-6, the job satisfaction checklist (Coefficient Alpha = .78) (Roessler & Rumrill, 1995a) was adapted from the Minnesota Theory of Work Adjustment developed by Dawis and Lofquist (1984). Respondents evaluate their satisfaction with their current jobs in terms of the twenty work reinforcers in the Minnesota theory. An example work reinforcer "I do things that make use of my abilities" may be responded to in one of three ways: (1) too little, (2) about right, or (3) too much. Respondents complete the section by listing two ways to make their jobs more personally satisfying. The changes identified may require discussing strategies for either decreasing or increasing the presence of a given reinforcer on the job.

Table 3-5. Assessing Job Mastery

Section IV. Job Mastery: Check (4) any concerns* that affect your success in completing the following tasks. Describe one solution for each of your two most important concerns.

1. Getting the job done
   - ✓ Believing that others think I do a good job.
   - ___Understanding how my job fits into the "big picture," i.e., the meaning of my job.
   - ___Knowing what I need to know to do my job.
   - ___Having what I need to do my job (knowledge, tools, supplies, equipment).

2. Fitting into the workforce
   - ✓ Scheduling and planning my work ahead of time.
   - ___Working mostly because I like the job.
   - ✓ Doing a good job.
   - ___Willing to make changes when necessary.

3. Learning the ropes
   - ___Knowing who to go to if I need help.
   - ___Understanding company rules and regulations.
   - ___Knowing my way around work.
   - ___Feeling a "part" of what is going on at work.

4. Getting along with others
   - ___Eating lunch with friends at work.
   - ___Having many friends at work.
   - ___Looking forward to seeing my friends at work.
   - ___Knowing what is expected of me socially on the job.

5. Getting ahead
   - ___Having a plan for where I want to be in my job in the future.
   - ___Understanding what I have to do to get promoted.
   - ___Knowing what training to complete to improve chances for promotion.
   - ___Talking with supervisor about what I need to do to get promoted.

6. Planning the next career step
   - ✓ Considering what I will do in the future.
   - ___Knowing what the opportunities are in this company.
   - ___Wanting to become more specialized in my job.
   - ___Having a good idea of how to advance in this company.

Describe one solution for each of your two most important job mastery concerns.

#1_____

#2_____

*Selected items from *The Career Mastery Inventory.* Used with permission of the author, John O. Crites, Crites Career Consultants, Boulder, Colorado.

Table 3-6. Assessing Job Satisfaction

Section V. Satisfaction*: Rate your current job on each of the following statements. Describe two ways to make your job more personally satisfying.

In my job ... (check one)	Too Little	About Right	Too Much
I do things that make use of my abilities.	✓	—	—
The job gives me a feeling of accomplishment.	✓	—	—
I am busy all the time.	—	—	✓
I can work alone on the job.	✓	—	—
I do something different every day.	—	—	✓
My pay compares well with that of other workers.	—	✓	—
The job provides for steady employment.	—	—	✓
The job has good working conditions.	✓	—	—
The job provides an opportunity for advancement.	✓	—	—
I get recognition for the work I do.	✓	—	—
I tell people what to do.	—	—	—
I am "somebody" in the community.	✓	—	—
My coworkers are easy to make friends with.	—	✓	—
I can do the work without feeling it is morally wrong.	—	✓	—
I can do things for other people.	—	—	✓
The company administers its policies fairly.	✓	—	—
My boss backs up the workers with top management.	✓	—	—
My boss trains the workers well.	—	—	—
I try out some of my ideas.	—	—	—
I make decisions on my own.	—	—	—

Describe two ways to make your job more personally satisfying.

#1_____

#2_____

*Work reinforcers from the Minnesota Theory of Work Adjustment. Dawis, R. & Lofquist, L. (1984). *A psychological theory of work adjustment.* Minneapolis: University of Minnesota.

Preparing an Accommodation Plan

To conclude the WES, respondents select their three highest priority barriers, suggest reasonable accommodations for those barriers, and indicate who could help implement reasonable accommodations and how they could help (see Table 3-7). The information collected in this section of the WES constitutes the essential elements of an accommodation plan that the person can share with his employer. In presenting information in the accommodation plan to the employer, the respondent should emphasize the relationship between barrier removal and increased productivity.

Table 3-7.   Developing an Accommodation Plan

Section VI. Review Sections II-V of the WES and list the three most significant barriers to success in your work. Describe their solutions and people/resources who can help. Be specific.

Barrier 1: _____
   Solution? _____

   _____

   _____

   Who can help? How can they help? _____

   _____

   _____

Barrier 2: _____
   Solution? _____

   _____

   _____

   Who can help? How can they help? _____

   _____

   _____

Barrier 3: _____
   Solution? _____

   _____

   _____

   Who can help? How can they help? _____

   _____

   _____

Administering the WES

Rehabilitation professionals may administer the WES in a face-to-face (Roessler & Gottcent, 1994) or telephone interview (Rumrill, Roessler, & Denny, in press) with individuals with disabilities who are either employed or about to begin employment. Whether conducted by telephone or in person, the WES interview requires thirty to sixty minutes to complete. Face-to-face contact enables the administrator to elicit more information from the respondent because it provides greater opportunity for feelings of trust to develop and for clarification of responses. Prior to administering the WES, rehabilitation professionals may wish to mentally "walk through" the interview using their own jobs as models.

The general procedure for completing WES Sections II through V is as follows:

1. Engage the person in identifying barriers to accessibility, performance of essential functions, job mastery, and job satisfaction.

2. Ask the person if any problems were overlooked, that is, not included in the checklist. If so, record the additional barriers in the appropriate section.

3. Encourage the person to suggest reasonable accommodations for the barriers; do not hesitate to share knowledge of accommodations that might prove feasible in the person's employment setting.

4. Help the person complete Section VI based on a thorough review of information in the preceding sections of the WES.

5. Remind the person that Section VI constitutes the basis for initiating a review of accommodation needs with the employer. It enables the person to state barriers to productivity in priority order, reasonable accommodation options for each barrier, and potential resources that could assist in barrier removal.

The WES administrator should make every effort to encourage respondents to elaborate on their impressions of their work environments, job duties, and barriers to their productivity. Such information is particularly useful when the rehabilitation professional is not familiar with the job that the person performs. For example, the WES administrator may not understand the details when a person states that she is an assembler. One respondent who worked on an assembly line used an air gun to place cover-boot wire around control panels on washing machines. Clearly, most WES administrators would need additional information to understand the demands of this task.

Respondents may also have difficulty discriminating between their job *titles* and their job *duties*. For example, a public school teacher needs to consider specific teaching functions and any barriers encountered in performing those functions. Essential functions of the teaching process include tasks such as reading, grading, talking/lecturing, writing, supervising children's activities, and attending faculty meetings. Even functions such as supervision and lecturing can be broken down into more specific tasks.

Throughout the administration of the WES, the interviewer should explain the meaning of any terms that are unfamiliar. For example, cognitive items in the essential functions section may require clarification. Respondents may question what temperature and ventilation have to do with accessibility. The interviewer should explain that excessive heat or cold or poor air circulation could influence one's breathing, which, in turn, affects mobility.

Some respondents have also requested clarification in responding to the section on job satisfaction (Section V). The administrator should instruct respondents to consider all items in relationship to the concept of job satisfaction. For example, in presenting the item "I do something different every day," the administrator should ask, "Are you satisfied with this?" If the respondent answers "yes," the correct answer is "about right." If the respondent says "no," the correct response is one that indicates dissatisfaction, that is, "too little" or "too much." The interviewer must probe to determine whether the person does "too little" or "too much" of the same thing every day.

Parts of the WES such as Sections II, III, and VI are helpful for unemployed people with MS who are planning to return to work. Information in the WES can help them identify suitable types of jobs and work environments and the assistive devices/accommodations they might need. They can also consider community agencies, technology resources, and employer-based services that are available to assist them in resuming work. Using the WES for prospective employment is basically a "needs" assessment, e.g., how accessible would the worksite have to be, how warm or cool would the work area have to be, could job duties involve walking long distances, what types of accommodations would be needed, and what resources are available.

The WES is also helpful for people with MS who have not disclosed their condition and have some discomfort about the prospect of disclosure. The WES can help them focus on concrete information, involve them in constructive problem-solving activities, and assist them in identifying appropriate people and agencies for resources. This type of focusing, and the resulting knowledge, may lessen their concerns about disclosure.

The Goldberg Scale

The Goldberg Scale addresses the theme of psychological uncertainty, which often stands as the greatest barrier to the resumption and retention of work for people with multiple sclerosis. Assessing the construct of vocational development, the Goldberg Scale measures problems encountered by people with disabilities that have a bearing on their motivation to work, realism, and rehabilitation outlook. This information is gathered by asking the respondent to answer a series of "semistructured questions that elicit a person's vocational plans, interests, work values, motivation to work, and rehabilitation outlook" (Goldberg, 1992, p. 167).

Administered in two stages, each interview requires approximately one hour to complete. Raters review the person's answers to arrive at an estimate of the individual's rehabilitation outlook, which includes motivation to return to work, a realistic assessment of capacities and physical limitations, and optimism about future recovery and rehabilitation after treatment.

Scores on the Goldberg Scale provide important insights into the probability that a person will successfully complete a rehabilitation program. People with a negative rehabilitation outlook have a low probability of success and experience feelings of hopelessness and devastation. Motivation to return to work, realistic assessment of capacities, and optimism are predictive of successful return to work. Because these factors play at least as important a role in resumption of employment as severity of disability, the rehabilitation professional should consider assessing and intervening in vocational development for individuals with

MS who have not succeeded in resuming or retaining employment.

Applications

The assessments presented in this chapter have many applications. First, they are extremely useful in the counseling relationship because they provide valuable information regarding both person and environment factors that affect vocational success. For example, data on work reinforcer preferences, vocational interests, type and seriousness of MS symptoms, and past work history are pertinent to determining whether a person will be successful in a current or prior line of work or whether she should pursue a related but different type of job. Information on rehabilitation outlook and self-care behaviors provides insights into the extent to which the person is likely to complete a rehabilitation program as well as to maintain a healthy lifestyle. Finally, findings regarding barriers in the work environment that require accommodation or modification are directly relevant to the person's chances to secure and retain desirable employment.

Findings from the assessments described in this chapter are useful to disability management professionals who seek to improve the employment-related services of their employers. Schwartz, Watson, Galvin, and Lipoff (1989, p. 1) defined disability management as the use of "services, people, and materials to (1) minimize the impact and cost of disability to employers and employees, and (2) encourage return to work for employees with disability." Information from assessments such as the WAS-I, WAS-E, and WES help employer and employee to collaborate in identifying barriers to productivity and cost-effective accommodations. Cost-effective (reasonable) accommodations can control rising workers' compensation and health care costs, which are consuming an increasing share of employer resources. One should also note that the assessments described in this chapter are not just for employees with multiple sclerosis or even other types of disabilities, but for other major segments of today's work force such as older workers. By gathering information pertinent to helping people care for themselves and remain productive at work, employers can retain trained workers during a time when decreasing numbers of workers with adequate skills are available in the labor market (McDaniel & Gysbers, 1992).

The Relevance of Assessments in the ADA Era

Information from assessments that identify factors affecting a person's capacity to do work are extremely relevant in the ADA era. Title I of the ADA describes employment protections that require accommodation of employees with disabilities so that they can perform essential job functions, provided that the accommodations do not constitute an undue hardship for the employer (Roessler & Rumrill, 1994a, 1995b). Data from the WAS-I, WAS-E, and WES are useful throughout the accommodation process prescribed by the ADA to resolve problems that people with MS face in performing their jobs. Feldblum (1991) described the steps of the accommodation process as follows:

1. The employee or applicant may initiate the request for an accommodation, to which the employer is required to respond.

2. The individual and the employer collaborate in a process of identifying the barriers that limit the worker's abilities to perform essential functions of the job.

3. Using the person with a disability as a source of information, the employer identifies a variety of accommodations.

4. The employer assesses the cost-effectiveness of each of the accommodations to determine which ones can be made with the least economic hardship to the business.

5. The employer implements the most appropriate accommodation with due consideration of the person's preferences in the case of two or more accommodations deemed equal in cost-effectiveness.

Information from the WES can help the employee understand specifically what her work limitations are, the priority to place on those limitations, and examples of reasonable accommodations. This information is useful throughout the five steps of the accommodation process. Moreover, the WES enables the employer to involve the person with a disability in the accommodation process, as Feldblum suggested in step three.

Assessment Data and Limiting the Intrusiveness of Disability

Ranging from measures of concrete constructs such as symptoms and daily living skills to more abstract concepts such as rehabilitation outlook, the assessments described in this chapter provide information regarding potentially helpful strategies to reduce the intrusiveness of multiple sclerosis and other severe disabilities. In addition to their physical effects, chronic illnesses and severe disabilities such as MS are intrusive psychosocial stressors that increase role strain, disrupt economic and vocational stability, and create a sense of helplessness and external control (Devins & Seland, 1987; Gecas, 1989). Understanding how MS has affected them can help people assume a more empowered role in the rehabilitation process. As a result, they gain a greater sense of self-efficacy, the belief that they have the power to achieve desirable outcomes and avoid negative ones (Bandura, 1986). Experiences that enhance self-efficacy are desirable antidotes to the negative impact of disability and chronic illness on personal control.

Summary

Several basic premises underlie this chapter on assessment of the employment needs of people with MS. For example, the strategy of least intervention may be the most sensible, i.e., assist the person in retaining employment in the same job with the same employer. If this is not possible, the person may initiate and direct his own vocational analysis with some assistance and identify related vocational roles that are available in the local job market. Occupational information resources such as the *Dictionary of Occupational Titles* and the *Occupational Outlook Handbook* are useful in this effort, as are specific assessments such as the Minnesota Importance Questionnaire (MIQ) and the Minnesota Satisfactoriness Scales (MSS).

Two other premises in the chapter work hand in hand, i.e., the concept of career development is more encompassing than simply functioning in vocational roles, and both person and environment must be assessed to identify appropriate vocational placements. Measures of symptoms associated with MS (the MS-RS) and factors impeding or enhancing the capacity to work at home, in the community, and in one's job (the ADL-MS, WAS-I, and WAS-E) operationalize a broader and more useful career construct. With information from these measures and other types of assessments such as job analyses, the rehabilitation professional can determine which person and environment interventions have the potential of maximizing the person's capacity to do work, i.e., expend energy to achieve personal goals in a wide range of settings.

By concentrating specifically on workplace barriers, the Work Experience Survey (WES) addresses the problem of excessively high unemployment rates among people with MS. The WES is based on the assumption that barriers may occur in four areas: access to the workplace, performance of essential functions, job mastery, and job satisfaction. Problems identified in any of the four areas are responsive to on-the-job adjustments ranging from the use of technology and other accommodative strategies to the changing of certain company policies or supervisory techniques. Suggested job accommodations and information as to who can assist the individual and how they can assist are organized in an accommodation plan in the final section of the WES.

Goldberg's measure of vocational development is useful for those individuals with MS who are having difficulty coping with the psychological uncertainty of the illness and its debilitating effects on the resumption and/or retention of employment. With its emphasis on motivation, realism, and optimism, the Goldberg Scale provides valuable insights into the person's rehabilitation outlook, a variable that research has shown to be related to work resumption. Scores on this scale may help the rehabilitation professional determine the types of psychological problems that the person is experiencing and the interventions that have the greatest potential to restore the person's motivation to continue employment.

Throughout all of the discussion of the various measurement strategies, the reader should keep in mind the broad applications related to the assessment of people with MS. Accurate assessment information on factors impeding and enhancing the production of work (defined broadly) can help (1) employers improve their disability management services, (2) people with MS participate in and benefit from the accommodation protections in the ADA, and (3) people with MS and their families take control of the rehabilitation and accommodation process in order to counter the helplessness and depression that are frequently experienced in cop-

Chapter 4

Job Placement and Retention Interventions

Phillip D. Rumrill, Jr.

The preceding chapters have established multiple sclerosis as one of the most common, unpredictable, and potentially debilitating neurologic disorders in the United States and other Western-block countries. The often severe medical and psychological accompaniments of this chronic disease may pose significant obstacles to functioning in virtually every aspect of life.

In considering the overall psychosocial impact of MS, the issue of employment warrants special recognition. Chapter 2 documented the multiplicity of demographic, psychological, medical, and social factors that can affect a person's career prospects following diagnosis, and it should be clear that the disappointing (25 percent) labor force participation rate among Americans with MS is not fully explained by the psychomedical effects of the illness. With this understanding of the wide-ranging and complex issues that affect employment following the onset of MS, the question for rehabilitation policymakers and practitioners alike becomes, "How can these issues be addressed in a way that removes or reduces the barriers to career success?"

For many Americans with disabilities, the answer to that question rests in the state-federal vocational rehabilitation (VR) program. Under the auspice and authority of Title I of the Rehabilitation Act of 1973 (and its subsequent amendments and reauthorizations), the Office of Special Education and Rehabilitative Services of the United States Department of Education annually administers more than two billion dollars to promote employment opportunities for people with severe disabilities (Rubin & Roessler, 1995). For people with MS, the key word in the previous sentence is "severe." Because funding for the VR program is insufficient to adequately meet the needs of the estimated 49 million disabled Americans, services are prioritized on

65

an "order of selection" basis that is predicated on the severity of the person's disability. In other words, VR counselors are charged with serving people with the most severe disabilities first and adding those with less severe impairments to caseloads only as funds permit.

To the extent that many symptoms of MS do not present "severe" functional limitations at any given point in time (Rumrill, 1993; Schapiro, 1994), people with MS do not utilize VR services to the same extent as those with other disabilities. In fact, LaRocca and Hall (1990) reported that only 806 people with MS were closed as "successful" VR clients in 1984—a number representing less than one percent of VR's successful case closures during that year.

Although the functional impact of MS does not, in most cases, warrant its designation as a "severe" disability within VR eligibility criteria, the fact remains that a high percentage of Americans with MS are unable to continue in their careers as the illness progresses. The need for proactive employment interventions can be directly inferred from the woeful post-diagnosis outcomes reported in Chapter 2. Specifically, rehabilitation professionals must consider ways to assist people with MS in both (1) seeking and securing jobs that are compatible with their interests and experiences, and (2) retaining jobs as the illness progresses. To that end, this chapter focuses on demonstrated placement and retention interventions that have the potential to increase labor force participation and success within the American MS community.

Job Placement Interventions

According to Rumrill (in press), rehabilitation practitioners working with people with MS must place a priority on assisting unemployed people in entering or re-entering the work force. In that endeavor, several strategies that have been reported in the professional literature are directly applicable to the far-reaching employment-assistance needs of people with MS. The following sections illustrate the primary tenets and relevant findings of four placement initiatives: MS Back-to-Work, the Job Raising Program, Return-to-Work, and the Career Possibilities Project.

MS Back-to-Work: Operation Job Match

In 1980, the National Capitol Chapter (Washington, D.C.) of the National Multiple Sclerosis Society instituted a job placement program for unemployed people with MS. The project, MS Back-to-Work (subsequently renamed Operation Job Match), was imbued with both job-seeking skills training and selective placement techniques such as those employed by vocational rehabilitation counselors in a wide range of service settings (Rubin & Roessler, 1995). The job-seeking skills component, which generally focuses on preparing the individual for an active role in the job acquisition process (Rubin & Roessler, 1995), included such topics as interviewing tips and etiquette and coping with on-the-job stress (LaRocca & Hall, 1990). Selective placement activities—interventions undertaken by the rehabilitation professional to facilitate placement opportunities for the person—included "matching" program participants with jobs identified through an MS-specific job bank (based on congruence between the interests of participants and the demands of particular positions). The job bank was formed by a network of corporate and small business sponsors who identified private-industry employment opportunities for people with MS (LaRocca, 1995).

MS Back-to-Work: Operation Job Match combined the best elements of the person-environment reciprocation that served as the conceptual basis for Chapter 3. It placed dual emphasis on increasing the job-seeking proficiency of participants and enlisting assistance from the employer community in generating a wide range of career options for people with MS. The success of the program in that endeavor led to its adoption and replication at numerous society chapters nationwide and as a constituent of the more comprehensive Job Raising program (LaRocca & Hall, 1990).

The Job Raising Program

In 1983, the National Multiple Sclerosis Society joined forces with the Arthritis Foundation and a consortium of advocacy groups representing people with traumatic brain injuries to develop the Job Raising Program—a placement and retention model for people with adult-onset, chronic disabilities. The Job Raising Program was conceived with the lofty aspiration of "greatly exceeding the success of any of the other existing rehabilitation-related programs, public or private" (Hall, 1991, p. 3).

Serving a total of 2,338 participants over the course of the eight-year project, the Job Raising Program provided a wide range of direct services. These services were delivered in a ten-week, small group (ten to twelve participants) format in which participants met for three hours once a week. Sharing the goal of obtaining and/or maintaining employment, participants received information and direction from community experts on such matters as (1) assertiveness, (2) interviewing skills, (3) resumé writing, and (4) the job market. Other employment-relevant issues included whether, how, and when to disclose one's disability to an employer; self-assessment strategies; and independent living (Hall, 1991). Following the ten-week process, participants formed a job search club as a means of staying in touch and supporting one another. They were also introduced to mentors who worked in their chosen fields.

The intensive and encompassing Job Raising Program proved to be a resounding success. Of the 2,338 people with MS, arthritis, and traumatic brain injuries who participated at thirty-nine sites nationwide, no fewer than 1,400 (60 percent) were employed eight years after the project's inception (Hall, 1991). Of particular relevance to this book is the fact that 71 percent of Job Raising participants who had MS were successfully employed at the eight-year follow-up. Other important outcomes of the project were as follows (Hall, 1991, p. 1):

1. It built the Job Raising model into one of the finest systems for empowering people with disabilities to maximize their choices for good jobs.

2. More than 1,250 separate employers throughout the country employ Job Raising participants.

3. Over 900 persons from the business community have contributed as advisory council members and/or mentors.

4. Thirty-nine sites spanning the entire country have fully implemented the program . . . during these eight years.

The most prominent feature of the Job Raising Program was its unique collaboration among disability groups, health care professionals, rehabilitation agencies, and employers. Its holistic approach serves as an exemplar of how to meet the complex employment needs of Americans with MS in a cost-effective and integrated fashion.

Return-to-Work

The fact that most people with MS have successful employment histories but leave their jobs within a few years of initial signs of the disease (LaRocca, 1995) means that placement interventions to assist unemployed people with the illness should be framed in a "return to work" context. Additionally, the support group model that serves as a service delivery mechanism for many programs offered by the National Multiple Sclerosis Society (see Chapter 7) must be viewed as a cost-effective and therapeutically sound alternative to individual counseling.

Perhaps the best combination of these emphases can be found in Roessler and Farley's (1993) Return-to-Work program (RTW). The RTW is a small-group intervention designed to encourage people with mid-career disabilities such as MS to re-enter the labor force. Intended as a post-acute, early-intervention strategy to assist people in overcoming such work disincentives as disability benefit (SSDI) restrictions and employer stereotypes regarding people with disabilities, the RTW applies rational emotive principles to motivate participants back to work.

According to Roessler (1988), the theoretical basis for RTW is a combination of systems theory and adult coping research. Systems theory holds that people strive to maintain homeostasis, or balance, in their lives (Shontz, 1975). Both having a disability such as MS and being unemployed interfere with that balance by threatening the person's inclination toward independence and self-control (Roessler, 1988). Consequently, people initiate coping responses to reduce stress and restore balance. The RTW provides a forum for people to develop effective coping strategies that reduce the stress associated with being unemployed. It challenges participants to develop "functional values, beliefs, and skills" that will guide them in the specific endeavor of returning to work and also in the general process of adjusting to and eventually accepting their disabilities. To the extent that employment is a common casualty of the early stages of MS, the RTW represents a logical mode of placement assistance and a sound personal adjustment experience. The three primary modules of the RTW—coping with disability and related life changes, life and benefits planning, and return to work—are detailed in the following paragraphs.

Module 1: Coping with Disability and Related Life Changes

In six-to-ten-person groups that spend approximately twenty-five hours in direct contact, RTW participants begin the process with an orientation and group cohesion exercises (Roessler & Farley, 1993). Following those introductory activities, RTW facilitators (typically rehabilitation professionals) engage participants in discussions of the impact that disability and unemployment have had on them. Specifically, participants examine the extent to which their emotional and behavioral reactions to disability have contributed to goal attainment, conflict resolution, and/or personal health and safety. As described in the *Return-to-Work Trainer's Manual* (Roessler & Farley, 1993), the specific activities included in Module 1 are as follows:

1. Return-to-Work (Introduction and Orientation)

2. Examples of Major Life Events

3. My Disability as a Major Life Event

4. Typical Reactions to Disability

5. My Reactions to My Disability

6. Changes in Major Life Areas

7. Determining If Emotions (Feelings) and Behaviors (Actions) Are in My Best Interest

8. My Reactions: Are They in My Best Interest?

9. Understanding Feelings and Actions

10. The Role of Beliefs

11. Major Beliefs About Events

12. Understanding Personal Reactions to Disability and Related Life Changes

13. How to Change Beliefs

14. Learning Rational Self-Statements

15. Practicing New Beliefs

Module 2: Life and Benefits Planning

In Chapter 2 of this book, disincentives in the Social Security program related to both income and health insurance were described as significant impediments to the full employment of people with MS (Keniston, 1995; LaRocca, 1995; Mahoney, 1995). Accordingly, any initiative to assist people with MS in resuming employment must include specific attention to the ways in which going back to work could affect the person's government benefits and other aspects of life planning.

In Module 2 of the RTW process, participants focus on how work fits into their long-term lifestyle plans. Roessler and Farley (1993) termed this step the "re-motivation phase of adjustment to mid-career disability." The dual emphasis on life planning and financial benefits includes such considerations as (1) the relative importance of and potential conflicts among various life roles (e.g., parent, spouse, worker, adult child, person with a disability, consumer of government services, household manager); (2) participants' readiness to adjust other roles to accommodate employment; (3) personal control mechanisms (influences) in the decision-making process; and (4) benefit systems and how they view paid employment. These issues are addressed in the small-group format to assist the participant in determining:

1. An overall goal with respect to work and life in general.

2. What additional information she needs to pursue that goal.

3. The impact that future events (such as the progression of MS) could have on attainment of that goal.

4. A list of alternative paths to consider in pursuing that goal.

5. Potential outcomes of each alternative (Roessler & Farley, 1993).

Before beginning the third module, RTW participants discuss financial concerns related to returning to work. For people with MS, these concerns may include retraining, child care, transportation, attendant care, medical treatment or therapy, costs associated with job-seeking activities, and assistive technology. Coupling these considerations with examination of benefit systems (noted previously), participants move to Module 3 with a clear picture of how rejoining the work force could affect their overall financial outlook. For people with MS and other disabilities, the financial risks of employment do not always outweigh the potential benefits (as described in depth in Chapter 6). Roessler and Farley (1993) suggested that RTW facilitators invite experts from the Social Security Administration to present information on selected work incentives in the SSI and SSDI programs. Appendix A presents selected resources and references concerning social security, workers' compensation, and long-term disability insurance (Roessler & Farley, 1993, pp. 78–79).

Module 3: Return-to-Work

The final module of the RTW program encourages participants to specify their vocational goals and begin the process of seeking and securing employment that is compatible with their interests, abilities, and experience. Activities include a graphic work readiness scale (Kanungo, 1982), an appraisal of the needs that would be met through employment (see Table 4–1), and an examination of preferred occupational titles and settings. Participants select at least two job alternatives to evaluate the "job/person match" (see Chapter 3) characteristics of each. In that evaluation, reasonable

Table 4-1. Meeting Needs Through Employment

Two attractive job choices:

1. _____

2. _____

Will this job help you. . .

	Job 1		Job 2	
	Yes	No	Yes	No
Make enough money?	____	____	____	____
Gain the respect of others?	____	____	____	____
Use your talents?	____	____	____	____
Make new friends?	____	____	____	____
Help other people?	____	____	____	____
Improve your skills?	____	____	____	____
Get control of your life?	____	____	____	____

accommodations (see Chapter 5) are discussed as means to enhance those "matches."

Module 3 culminates with the formulation of a vocational goal plan for each participant to implement. Each person selects a specific job to pursue and specifies services and personal actions required to complete her employment plan. An employment expectation—ranging from unemployment to full-time employment—is projected for each of three "checkpoints": three months, six months, and one year after completion of the RTW program. The final job goal is stated in terms of the steps that the participant will take (in sequence) to attain that goal (Roessler & Farley, 1993).

Following completion of Module 3, RTW participants return for regular follow-up sessions (at time intervals determined by facilitators and group members) to discuss their progress. Group support, discussion of successes and problems in the job-seeking process, and adjustments of participants' goal plans (if needed) are key elements of these sessions. Roessler and Farley (1993) advised RTW facilitators to continue this monitoring for three to six months.

The mid-career nature of MS makes the Return-to-Work program an ideal placement strategy for people with the illness who wish to re-enter the labor force. Delivered in an efficient group format, the RTW affords participants the opportunity to benefit from one another's insights and experiences as they progress through the career re-motivation and re-initiation processes together. Content-area considerations such as the impact of employment on disability benefits and the importance of on-the-job accommodations round out the utility of the RTW as a timely and appropriate intervention for members of the MS community.

The Career Possibilities Project

In 1994, the Arkansas Research and Training Center in Vocational Rehabilitation (University of Arkansas) received a Health Services Research grant from the National Multiple Sclerosis Society to develop, demonstrate, and evaluate the Career Possibilities Project. Addressing LaRocca's (1995) call for empowerment, rights awareness, resource utilization, and community-based services as research priorities concerning MS and employment, the project targeted unemployed people with MS at four sites across the midwestern United States: Cleveland, Ohio; Evansville, Indiana;

Louisville, Kentucky; and Milwaukee, Wisconsin. The primary purpose of the study was to increase participants' (1) placement rate, (2) job-seeking activity, (3) employability maturity, (4) optimism about re-entering the work force, and (5) career self-efficacy.

Utilizing a two-group, pretest/posttest quasi-experimental design, project investigators (Drs. Richard Roessler and Phillip Rumrill) recruited fifty participants from MS Society chapters and MS clinics in the four cities listed previously. Using time sampling methods, researchers assigned the first twenty-five participants to the Career Possibilities condition. The second twenty-five participants to volunteer for the study were assigned to the comparison group.

The twenty-five participants in the comparison group completed a telephone interview with a trained rehabilitation professional about their job-seeking plans and received written job-seeking information. The information packet contained tips and strategies for securing job leads, developing resumés, interviewing, following up after interviews, and networking. This limited intervention was compared to the more elaborate and resource-based Career Possibilities condition.

The Career Possibilities intervention involved (1) a telephone interview with a trained rehabilitation professional concerning the participant's career interests and experiences; and (2) a resource-utilization seminar that introduced her to an employer in her chosen field and a rehabilitation professional to facilitate the career re-entry process.

The Accommodations Planning Team (APT) seminar served as the basis for the Career Possibilities intervention. The APT is a half-day program that enables people with disabilities to (1) identify their prospective needs for on-the-job accommodations; (2) understand their legal rights to reasonable accommodations; (3) discuss their accommodation needs with employers in their career fields; and (4) develop resource-directed plans for obtaining career-entry or re-entry positions (Rumrill, Roessler, Boen, & Brown, 1995). The following paragraphs describe the APT format and component activities in detail (Reed, Rumrill, Roessler, Brown, & Boen, 1994; Rumrill, Roessler, Boen, & Brown, 1995).

Introduction

Before the APT seminar begins, it is helpful to provide an orientation to the program for participating job-seekers. Before they meet their teams, APT participants receive verbal information about what the seminar will entail and a copy of the program agenda (see Table 4–2). Then, as a prelude to team activities, participants receive tips on interviewing and self-presentation, including appropriate dress, interviewing etiquette, and commonly asked interview questions. When participants are introduced to their teams at the beginning of the APT seminar, participants and employers are asked to simulate an abbreviated job interview as a means of introduction. The third member of each team, a rehabilitation professional, observes the introductory interview and offers constructive feedback.

Identifying Job-Specific Accommodation Needs

Once introductions and simulated interviews have been completed, the first step in the APT seminar involves helping the participant identify her prospective needs for job accommodations. The preliminary telephone interview helps the person with MS to specify his career re-entry goal, and the needs identification phase of the APT seminar engages him in a process of considering how attainment of that goal could be facilitated by identifying and removing any disability-related barriers on that particular job. Job accommodations include those modifications and aids that enable an individual with a disability to perform the essential functions of a job (Equal Employment Opportunity Commission & Department of Justice, 1991; see Chapter 5).

In the APT seminar, the Work Experience Survey (WES) (Roessler, 1995) is used to assist participants in identifying both disability-related barriers to productivity on the job and reasonable accommodations that could assist them in overcoming those barriers. Although the WES consists of six sections, APT participants complete only Sections II, III, and VI. Respectively, these sections address accessibility (getting to, from, and around on the job), essential job functions (problems with specific job demands or working conditions), and the accommodation plan (the participant's three most important employment barriers, feasible accommodations, and possible resources).

Guided by seminar facilitators who are trained rehabilitation professionals, participants begin the needs identification process by considering a list of twenty possible barriers to worksite

Table 4-2.   Accommodating Planning Team (APT) Seminar Agenda

1:00 P.M.	Interview Skills Training Dressing for success Communication skills Job search etiquette Questions all employers ask Questions about disability and disclosure
2:00 P.M.	Introduction to APT and Simulated Interviews Welcome and overview Practice interviews—employers/applicants Feedback from rehabilitation professionals
2:30 P.M.	Identifying Accommodation Needs The Work Experience Survey Barriers, solutions, and resources A team approach to accommodation planning
3:10 P.M.	The Americans with Disabilities Act (ADA) Title I definitions and regulations Consumer rights and responsibilities Employer obligations Disclosure Collaborating to implement accommodations
3:30 P.M.	Discussing Accommodations with Your Employer The "Win-Win" approach Communication: The key to success Employer/applicant accommodation discussion Feedback from rehabilitation professionals
4:00 P.M.	Placement Planning: Restarting Your Career Where to look and who can help Widening your options Follow-up contacts: Be persistent A team approach to step-by-step planning
4:30 P.M.	Social Security Work Incentives Overview Where to get assistance
4:45 P.M.	Reflections on the APT Process Applicant's next steps Conclusion and program evaluation

accessibility. These include parking, entrance, floors/floor coverings, lighting, evacuation routes, and ventilation. Using the employer's place of business as an example, team members indicate which of the twenty accessibility items could present a problem for the participant. After determining whether any other barriers might exist, teams "brainstorm" possible solutions to the two most important accessibility barriers. A technology specialist from the Division of Vocational Rehabilitation services or a community agency is also available during the APT seminar to provide additional consultation.

In Section III of the WES, APT participants identify any job demands or conditions (related to essential job functions) that might pose barriers. As described in Chapter 3, the essential functions section includes six categories: physical abilities, cognitive abilities, task-related abilities, social abilities, working conditions, and company policies. Again, employers and rehabilitation professionals provide valuable assistance by clarifying the requirements and working conditions in the participants' chosen fields. The technology specialist is available during this phase to suggest types of job accommodations (both high and low tech) that would meet participants' needs.

Having identified accessibility (Section II) and essential function (Section III) barriers and solutions, participants solicit team recommendations for the accommodation plan (Section VI). The plan specifies the participant's top three barriers, feasible solutions for each, and resources that can help her with implementing accommodations. Once again, the employer, rehabilitation professional, and technology specialist serve as consultants to the participant. Ideas on the accommodation plan are utilized during the final phase of the APT seminar—formulation of a placement plan. Before developing a placement plan, however, the participant is provided with in-depth information concerning (1) the employment (Title I) provisions of the ADA, and (2) effective strategies for approaching an employer to request a reasonable accommodation.

Understanding the ADA's Key Terms and Employment Protections

Once participants have identified their prospective needs for on-the-job accommodations via the WES, the next step in the

APT seminar format involves understanding their rights to employment accommodations under the ADA. In this phase, facilitators outline the key terms and provisions of the ADA, focusing on Title I (Employment). Specifically, participants are informed that the ADA:

1. Provides civil rights protection for people with disabilities in broad areas of social activity, including employment.

2. Prohibits employment discrimination on the basis of disability.

3. Requires most public and private employers to provide reasonable accommodations that allow qualified people with disabilities to perform essential job functions.

4. Prevents employers from asking disability-related questions on application forms or at job interviews.

5. Requires the applicant or employee to disclose his or her disability before becoming eligible for reasonable accommodations.

6. Requires employers and employees to work together to identify and implement accommodations.

7. Provides specific legal remedies for persons who have been discriminated against (Rumrill, Roessler, Boen, & Brown, 1995, p. 97).

APT participants also receive detailed information concerning the key definitions and specific provisions of Title I—as will be covered in depth in Chapter 5. Understanding those provisions and definitions will help the participant to request needed accommodations from a prospective or current employer. Following the identification of needs and ADA information, APT teams convene to assist participants in practicing the self-presentation and communication skills they will need to secure career re-entry positions and to accommodate MS-related limitations on those jobs.

Developing Effective Self-Presentation Strategies

The next phase of the APT seminar is a role play activity between the participant and the employer on her team. Guided by seminar facilitators and observed by the rehabilitation professional, role play gives the participant the opportunity to practice discussing her experiences, credentials, and needs for on-the-job accommodations. The following guidelines (Rumrill, Roessler,

Boen, & Brown, 1995, p. 98) help the participant bring a tone of collaboration and mutual benefit to the discussion:

1. Use your top three accommodation needs from the WES as bases for discussion.

2. Discuss your disability only in terms of the limitations it presents.

3. Emphasize how reasonable accommodations will make you a more productive employee.

4. Use collaborative language (e.g., "Together we could. . . ," "It makes sense for both of us to. . ."), rather than adversarial or accusatory terms (e.g., "The law says you have to. . . ," "You can't discriminate against me. . .").

5. With the employer, generate solutions that meet each of your accommodation needs. Share your ideas about resources (e.g., vocational rehabilitation counselors) who can facilitate the accommodation process.

6. End the meeting with an agreement as to which accommodations will be provided and when they will be implemented.

7. Remember that many accommodations cost nothing or very little to implement. The ADA requires that accommodations be *reasonable*, but that does not mean that your accommodations must be of optimal benefit. The employer does make the decision as to which accommodations will be provided, but you do have the right to appeal.

After the role play has been completed, APT facilitators ask each rehabilitation professional to offer feedback on the participant's performance. Team members emphasize the positive aspects of the participant's presentation, framing corrective feedback in terms of suggestions for improvement rather than criticism.

Formulating Goal-Directed Placement Plans for Job-Seeking and Accommodation Activities

The final phase of the APT seminar involves specification of the participants' job-seeking plans. Incorporating information from the needs assessment, ADA awareness, and role play phases, teams assist their participants to identify employers who might be hiring and consider resources that can facilitate the job search process. The placement plan takes the form of a written, step-by-step guide that participants can use as a reference throughout the job search process (see Table 4–3). APT facilitators introduce the placement plan phase of the seminar with the following job-seeking tips:

1. Identify jobs of interest. Consult the following resources: (a) *Dictionary of Occupational Titles*, (b) *Guide for Occupational Exploration*, and (c) *Occupational Outlook Handbook*.

2. Learn where the jobs exist. This information may come from: (a) family and friends, (b) placement offices, (c) professional listing services, (d) newspapers (classifieds and articles), (e) professional journals and newsletters, (f) Chambers of Commerce, (g) telephone books, (h) State Employment Security Division job services, (i) vocational rehabilitation placement specialists, (j) job fairs, (k) civic organizations, and (l) APT seminar team members.

3. Contact (via telephone, letters, and in-person visits) all employers you can identify in your field. Even if they are not presently hiring, they may be in the near future. Meet them in person whenever possible.

4. Follow up all contacts with thank you letters or phone calls.

5. Be persistent. Getting a good job can be a full-time occupation in itself. Don't get discouraged, and keep following up on your contacts.

6. Remember your resources as the job search continues. Keep in regular contact with anyone who might help you find a position.

7. Finally, keep in mind your rights to reasonable accommodations under the ADA. Don't let your disability limit your options (Rumrill, Roessler, Boen, & Brown, 1995, p. 99).

After participants' plans for post-seminar job-seeking have been specified, APT facilitators ask each participant to share his or her career goals and intended placement activities with the group. Public commitment to a task is a documented antecedent of performance (Kanfer & Goldstein, 1991), and participants who share their plans will be more likely to follow through on them. The APT seminar concludes with one member of each team volunteering to contact the participant in two to four weeks as a follow-up measure. Facilitators may wish to end the program with a lunch or dinner. The meal provides a forum for informal dis-

Table 4-3.

WRITTEN PLACEMENT PLAN

NAME_____

CAREER GOAL(S)_____

_____

_____

GEOGRAPHIC AREAS OF FOCUS_____

_____

_____

_____

WHO CAN HELP?

NAME/TITLE	AFFILIATION/ ADDRESS	PHONE #	REFERRAL SOURCE	CONTACT DATE	CONTACT RESULT

Next Steps

1.   4.

2.   5.

3.   6.

cussion, and it offers an opportunity for a motivational "send-off" to the entire group. In past seminars, that address has been delivered by community leaders who happen to have MS, APT facilitators, and APT team members.

In numerous applications with several samples of people with disabilities, the APT seminar has proven to be an effective placement strategy that introduces the participant to valuable community resources and offers timely information concerning the ADA's accommodation process. Preliminary results of the Career Possibilities Project suggest that the seminar increases (1) confidence in the job search process, (2) the frequency of job-seeking activities, and (3) optimism about future career prospects among unemployed people with MS.

Although each of the job placement programs presented in the preceding sections is distinct in its scope and specific orientation, they all share consideration of the personal, social, and task-related factors that can impinge on career development for people with MS. They are imbued with the person-environment interaction illustrated by Dr. Richard Roessler in Chapter 3, and they address the myriad of concerns that can confront a person who is trying to re-establish his or her career while coping with a serious illness such as MS. Readers are reminded that the emphasis of any job placement program should be people's interests, abilities, and experience—not their disabilities and accompanying limitations.

Job Retention Interventions

In keeping with the person-environment orientation of Chapter 3, Roessler and Rumrill (1994a) exhorted rehabilitation professionals to accompany job placement services with early-intervention strategies designed to assist employed people with MS to maintain their careers. Crites (1976) theorized that a person's prospects for career adjustment and long-term success depend largely on his ability to overcome thwarting conditions, or barriers, in the world of work. The career maintenance barriers that result from MS were described in detail in Chapter 2, and their range and severity underscore the need for proactive interventions that enhance people's ability to overcome MS-related obstacles that they encounter on the rungs of the career ladder. The following sections describe two such job retention interventions, the Progressive Request Model and Project Alliance.

The Progressive Request Model

In a recent experimental investigation, Rumrill, Roessler, and Denny (in press) demonstrated the Progressive Request Model, an intervention wherein forty-five employed people with MS received varying levels of information and skill training concerning the ADA's employment accommodation process. Participants were "blocked" into groups of three according to similarities in (1) gender, (2) duration of illness, and (3) occupational type.

Within these blocks, they were then randomly assigned to one of three treatment conditions—control, prompt, or Progressive Request Model (PRM). Fifteen participants were included in each group.

The pure control condition involved no intervention. Control participants in the post-only study completed several outcome measures eight weeks after the prompt and PRM interventions had been concluded. The prompt condition included administration of the WES in a face-to-face interview coupled with a verbal prompt that participants approach their employers about their needs for reasonable accommodations. The more elaborate PRM intervention (Rumrill, 1993; Rumrill, Roessler, & Denny, in press; see Table 4–4) consisted of the WES, an ADA self-help guide (*Enhancing Productivity on Your Job: The "Win-Win" Approach to Reasonable Accommodations*; Roessler & Rumrill, 1994a, 1995b), and social competence training on how to effectively and assertively request accommodations from one's employer.

Table 4-4. Steps of the Progressive Request Model Intervention

Progressive Request Model (PRM) participants will receive an intervention consisting of (a) the Work Experience Survey, (b) a booklet describing the ADA's Title I procedures and provisions, and (c) a short, behavioral accommodation orientation program. PRM procedures should go as follows:

1. Telephone participants and ask for a 30–40 minute appointment at their homes to complete the Work Experience Survey (WES) interview. The appointment should be scheduled within the next 7–10 days.

2. After PRM participants have completed the WES home interviews, give them a copy of the ADA booklet. Discuss the purpose of the publication (provide a brief overview of its contents). Ask them to read it carefully, and ask if you can come back to their homes in one week to discuss the booklet's contents. Tell them that the next visit will take approximately one hour.

3. The second home visit will consist of a review of the booklet's contents, followed by a short training program designed to help PRM participants request accommodation reviews by their employers. Take about 15 minutes to review the booklet, and answer any questions the participant might have about its contents. Then, refer to the "win-win" discussion strategies.

4. The PRM program was designed to help participants develop and practice strategies for discussing their on-the-job needs with employers. Steps of the 45-minute accommodations orientation include:

Table 4-4. (*continued*)

a. Read the tips from the booklet aloud to participants. Answer any of their preliminary questions.

b. Ask the participant to play the part of the employer, and model an appropriate, collaborative ("win-win") discussion (5–10 minutes). Demonstrate appropriate introduction, basic courtesies (shaking hands, waiting to be asked before you sit, etc.), body language, verbal language, and the "win-win" negotiation strategies that are presented in the booklet.

c. Discuss the behaviors you model and their appropriateness for (generalizability) the participant's employer. Ask participants to suggest how your demonstration might be modified to meet their particular needs. For example, ask participants how their employers would receive your presentation, and generate with them techniques for maximizing the employers' receptivity.

d. Switch roles. Ask the participant to initiate a discussion of accommodation needs, and you serve as the employer. From the information already provided about the participant's employer, try to project an accurate representation of how the employer might react. For the first rehearsal, try to present a reasonably receptive employer. Be understanding, present some knowledge of how to accommodate persons with disabilities, and show a sincere but realistic interest in accommodating the participant's needs.

e. Provide feedback on the first "trial run." Emphasize the positive elements of the participant's presentation first. Frame constructive criticism in terms of making the presentation even more effective (__ , __ , and were excellent, and you could communicate even better by __ and __.").

f. Ask the participant to demonstrate the request and discussion process one more time, incorporating the feedback from the first trial. Present a slightly less receptive employer this time, one who is more interested in the bottom line—"What good will this do the company?", "What will all this cost me?"—than in accommodating someone's needs. The employer in the second practice meeting should know very little about the needs of workers with disabilities and be more or less indifferent to providing accommodations. Do not respond in a negative, confrontational, or rude manner, but do make the participant present his needs and the "win-win" nature of reasonable situations.

g. Provide feedback and discuss the second trial with the participant. Explain that most employers will be more cooperative than you were, but that you wanted to prepare them for a less than supportive response.

h. Remind the participant of the "What if . . .?" contingency—what to do in the event of employer discrimination. Refer to the booklet for specific recourses.

i. Review the "win-win" process a final time from beginning to end. Encourage the participant to initiate discussion with his or her employer as soon as possible. Indicate that you expect to hear that he or she has met with the employer in the very near future. Tell the participant that you will call back in eight weeks for information about the results of his or her discussion.

At an eight-week follow-up, Rumrill, Roessler, and Denny (in press) hypothesized that control, prompt, and PRM participants would perform in ascending order on (1) career maintenance self-efficacy (confidence in requesting reasonable accommodations), (2) acceptance of disability, (3) requests for accommodations made with employers, (4) meetings with employers to discuss reasonable accommodations, and (5) accommodations implemented at the worksite. Results upheld the hypothesized direction of career maintenance self-efficacy scores; PRM participants were significantly more confident in their abilities to advocate for themselves than were either prompt or control participants. Between-group differences on the behavioral measures (requests, meetings, and implemented accommodations) followed the predicted direction but were not significant at the .05 probability level. The intervention had no effect on global measures of acceptance of disability.

In speculating as to why increased self-efficacy (confidence) in the ADA's accommodation request process was not an antecedent of the specific behaviors that are prescribed, Rumrill, Roessler, and Denny (in press) suggested that their micro-skills approach to self-advocacy could have limited the effectiveness of the intervention. They stressed the need for employer involvement in accommodation planning, stating, "By involving the employer in the WES interview and offering ADA information and 'win-win' training to both parties, future career maintenance researchers can actively involve the employee's environment in the accommodation process." (Rumrill, Roessler, & Denny, in press, p. 13).

Project Alliance: Integrating Comprehensive Job Analysis Techniques and Employer Consultation

Findings presented by Rumrill, Roessler, and Denny (in press) underscore the importance of employer involvement in comprehensive job retention interventions. To the extent that reasonable accommodations are cost-effective (Berkeley Planning Associates, 1982) and often easy to implement (Roessler & Rumrill, 1995a), both employee and employer can benefit from consultation and technical assistance concerning strategies to overcome the employee's MS-related work limitations.

In 1992, the National Multiple Sclerosis Society introduced Project Alliance, "perhaps the crowning achievement of the Society in regard to employment" (LaRocca, 1995, p. 33). Combining needs assessment principles (Roessler, 1995) and self-advocacy training for employees (Rumrill, 1994; Rumrill, Roessler, & Denny, in press), Project Alliance added consultation with employers and the involvement of community resources in its full spectrum of job retention services (Sumner, 1995).

Available to employed (full- or part-time) people with MS and other chronic illnesses at fourteen sites nationwide, Project Alliance served more than three hundred employees (and their employers). The primary objectives of this comprehensive and collaborative program were as follows:

1. To engage both the employee (with a chronic illness) and the employer in the process of examining the current issues related to job performance.

2. To gather information related to the person's actual position, including the physical and cognitive requirements, the essential and marginal functions, and support systems.

3. To identify barriers to successful job performance.

4. To provide assistance to the employee and the employer in improving communication and in moving toward satisfactory resolution of the (work-related) issues.

5. To assist all parties in understanding the provisions of the ADA and how voluntary compliance can benefit all concerned.

6. To help identify needs of the employee and employer in terms of job modifications, adjustments, or accommodations that could assist the employee in achieving and maintaining satisfactory work performance (Sumner, 1995, p. 1).

The essence of the Project Alliance intervention was an on-site job analysis conducted by a trained rehabilitation professional. Gathering data from the employee with MS or other chronic illness, his employer, and coworkers, the job analyst recorded and interpreted such information as (1) the essential and marginal functions of the employee's position, (2) the employee's general and illness-related health status, (3) the impact of the illness on the employee's job performance, (4) the quality and quantity of the employee's work in comparison to his colleagues, (5) on-the-job and community resources that could be consulted, and (6) employee and employer appraisals of the presenting problem(s). The job analyst synthesized that information in a report presented to both the employee and the employer. Then, the job analyst made follow-along contacts for the next several weeks to assist in the implementation of reasonable accommodations and in consultation with recommended community resources.

As is detailed in Chapter 5, Title I of the ADA requires the employee with a disability and her employer to collaborate in a process of identifying, prioritizing, and implementing reasonable accommodations that enable the employee to perform the essential functions of her position. With its emphasis on "win-win" communication and mutually beneficial solutions to the disability-related barriers that confront people with MS at the workplace, Project Alliance exemplified the ADA's spirit of collaborative decision-making and non-adversarial problem-solving. It also served to educate employers concerning the benefits of retaining experienced and productive employees via reasonable accommodations.

Summary

People with MS may not utilize VR services to the same extent as people with other types of disabilities, but assistance is available! As is noted in Chapter 7, many chapters of the National Multiple Sclerosis Society have participated in initiatives designed to promote career opportunities for Society members. These initiatives have included Operation Job Match, the Job Raising Program, the Career Possibilities Project, the Progressive Request Model, and Project Alliance—and the Return-to-Work model features a group approach to career re-entry that is highly compatible with the Society's mission of helping others while helping oneself.

Unfortunately, this author's predominant use of the past tense in describing these programs reflects the fact that most were adopted as time-limited, demonstration projects. Efforts to incorporate these interventions into existing service delivery models must continue. Readers are encouraged to contact the author or their local Society chapters for additional information concerning job placement and/or retention assistance.

Chapter 5

Employment and the Americans with Disabilities Act: Civil Rights and Beyond

Phillip D. Rumrill, Jr.

In 1990, President George Bush signed into law the Americans with Disabilities Act (ADA), the first major article of civil rights legislation for people with disabilities. Mirroring the tenets of the Civil Rights Act of 1964, the five titles of the ADA provide antidiscrimination protection and equal access to employment opportunities, public services, public accommodations, and communication systems. Enactment of the ADA extended responsibility for accommodating people with disabilities to the private sector, which, except for government contractors, had been exempt from such disability legislation as the Rehabilitation Act of 1973.

Title I of the ADA provides employment protection for Americans with disabilities. It compels both private and public entities to establish and maintain nondiscriminatory hiring practices. Perhaps most importantly, it requires employers to provide reasonable accommodations that enable otherwise qualified people with disabilities to perform the essential functions of their jobs (Equal Employment Opportunity Commission & Department of Justice, 1991).

Introduced and enacted on the strength of efforts by consumer groups within the disability community (including the National Multiple Sclerosis Society) (Shapiro, 1993), the ADA emphasizes consumer participation in every aspect of the implementation process (Rumrill, 1993, 1994; Rumrill et al., 1995, in press). In fact, the ADA is so committed to individual privacy and consumer initiation of information that it precludes covered employers from asking disability-related questions on application forms or during job interviews, thereby requiring the person to disclose his disability as the initial step in the accommodation process.

Title I of the ADA provides comprehensive protection for people with disabilities at all levels and stages of employment, but its consumer-involvement mandates make it necessary for consumers to be keenly aware of their rights to nondiscriminatory treatment and procedures for invoking them. Unfortunately, studies have shown that most people with multiple sclerosis know very little about the ADA (Sumner, 1995), and that they lack confidence in their ability to advocate for themselves in employment (Rumrill, 1993; Rumrill, Roessler, & Denny, in press). Hence, they tend not to avail themselves of such strategies as reasonable accommodations that might enable them to continue working (Duggan, Fagan, & Yateman, 1993),

Indeed, LaRocca (1995, pp. 5–6) advised, "more education programs are needed to inform people with MS about such matters as their legal rights and job accommodations. . . . A proactive approach is [also] needed to maximize utilization of the Americans with Disabilities Act . . . and other legislation since people with MS seem to underutilize these opportunities." Accordingly, the purpose of this chapter is to provide "plain English" information concerning Title I of the ADA and its relevance to people with MS. Unless otherwise noted, the information to follow has been excerpted from *Enhancing Productivity on Your Job: The "Win-Win" Approach to Reasonable Accommodations* (Roessler & Rumrill, 1994a, 1995b), a Title I guide for people with MS sponsored by a Health Services Research grant from the National Multiple Sclerosis Society and reprinted herein with the kind permission of the Society.

Enhancing Productivity on Your Job: The "Win-Win" Approach to Reasonable Accommodations

Introduction

Enhancing Productivity on Your Job is written for you if you are currently employed or looking for a job and have a diagnosis of MS. Should problems related to your MS affect your job performance, you will need to identify job modifications—called "accommodations" in legal language—that will enable you to continue doing your job. The best argument for changing the way you do your job and/or the equipment you need to do it is to show that these accommodations will help you maintain your productivity level or become an even more productive employee.

Because everyone wins when employees maintain and enhance their productivity, we stress the importance of a "win-win" collaborative approach in discussing job accommodations with your employer. The "win-win" approach is much more likely to produce cooperative solutions to your on-the-job needs than is a legal procedure. It is also more likely to encourage a positive long-term working relationship with your employer.

Although we highly recommend this approach, we recognize that some employers may not respond to your needs for an accommodation review or for a satisfactory accommodation. We also recognize the risks involved in disclosing that you have a disability, which you must do to request an accommodation. Therefore, you first need to know your legal rights under the ADA.

Before You Begin: Know Your Rights

Because it is an informal, collaborative process, the "win-win" approach does not require any legal assertion of your rights. It is essential, however, that you know your rights, responsibilities, and potential risks before beginning this process. These facts about the employment provisions of the ADA will help you participate as a knowledgeable and confident "win-win" strategist.

What Is the ADA All About?

The ADA provides civil rights protection for people with disabilities in areas that are parallel to those established by the federal government on behalf of women and minorities (in the Civil Rights Act of 1964). One of the key provisions is Title I, the employment section, which requires employers to discuss your needs for on-the-job accommodations and to help you secure "reasonable accommodations."

You are covered by Title I of the ADA if (1) you have a disability (such as MS), have a record of having a disability, or are perceived as having a disability; (2) you meet the employer's requirements for a job; and (3) you have the capabilities to perform the essential functions of your current job or a job for which you wish to apply (with reasonable accommodations, if needed).

Employers and the ADA

Apart from employers with fewer than fifteen employees, the federal government, native American tribes, and tax-exempt private membership clubs, all employers must comply with Title I of the ADA. Sections 501-504 of the Rehabilitation Act of 1973 prevent the federal government, federal contractors, and any programs receiving federal funds from discriminating against people with disabilities.

What Does the ADA Prohibit?

Simply put, Title I of the ADA prohibits discrimination in employment against otherwise qualified people with disabilities. Here are some key definitions you should know:

Disability: Physical or mental impairment that substantially limits one or more major life activities such as walking, seeing, hearing, speaking, learning, and working.

Qualified: A person who satisfies the primary qualifications for a position and who can perform the essential functions of the job, with or without reasonable accommodations.

Essential functions: Primary job duties, as opposed to marginal duties, that the person must be capable of performing, with or without reasonable accommodations. Essential functions may be established by a job analysis and should be included in the written job description given to all prospective employees and all current workers who request one.

A function is considered essential if (1) the position primarily exists to perform the function, (2) there is a limited number of employees who can perform the function, and/or (3) the function is so specialized that the person is hired for his ability to perform it. Specific factors that enter into essential function determinations include (1) the employer's judgment, (2) the amount of time spent performing the function, (3) the consequences of not performing the function, (4) the terms of a collective bargaining agreement, (5) the work experience of past employees in that job, and (6) the work experience of current employees in similar jobs (Rumrill, Mullins, Hartshorn, & Reed, 1994).

Why the ADA?

You should be judged on your ability to do the job, not on stereotypes about a certain diagnosis or on fears about a certain disability. Multiple sclerosis may cause changes in your capacities over time, but there are ways to adjust for many of those changes. Furthermore, you have the legal right to a reasonable accommodation. Employers who are covered under Title I are required to consider and accommodate your MS-related needs.

These accommodations must be reasonable and not cause undue hardship for the employer. Two key phrases require more discussion: "reasonable accommodation" and "undue hardship."

What Is a "Reasonable Accommodation?"

An accommodation is a modification to the work environment or to the way an essential job function is performed. The purpose of the accommodation is to allow an otherwise qualified person to enter or continue in employment by removing significant disability-related work limitations.

Significant work limitations occur when problems related to your MS interfere with your abilities. For example, you may find that your work station is located too far from other areas in which you are required to work. Physical barriers such as flights of stairs or slippery floor coverings may impede your movement about the workplace. You may have problems with the equipment you must operate or the conditions under which you must operate it; for example, noise or vibration levels, temperature variations, or fumes that bother you. Finally, you may encounter certain job functions with physical requirements that constitute hazards to you or to others; for example, lifting or moving heavy objects. The ADA describes nine remedies for on-the-job barriers. They are (Roessler, Rumrill, & Reed, 1995):

▲ Restructuring of existing facilities
▲ Restructuring of the job

▲ Modification of work schedules

▲ Reassignment to another position

▲ Modification of equipment

▲ Installation of new equipment

▲ Provision of qualified readers and interpreters

▲ Modification of application and examination procedures and training materials

▲ Flexible personal leave policies

The following paragraphs provide descriptions and examples of each category. Much of the material is based on the ADA Handbook (Equal Employment Opportunity Commission & Department of Justice, 1991).

Restructuring of Existing Facilities

One of the primary requirements of Title I is that the work environment must be accessible. All facilities that are or will be used by an applicant or employee with a disability must be reasonably modified to accommodate the person's individual needs. This does not imply, however, that all facilities must be entirely accessible to all people with disabilities. Title I regulations make it very clear that reasonable accommodations are to be considered on an individual, case-by-case basis. The following are examples of how existing facilities can be restructured to create accessible work environments:

▲ Installation of a wheelchair ramp at the entrance of a building

▲ Installation of an electric door opener

▲ Reservation of widened parking spaces for wheelchair users

▲ Renovation of restrooms

▲ Installation of handrails and textured detectable warnings on stairways for people with visual impairments

Restructuring of the Job

A job may be restructured for an employee with a disability if the restructuring involves marginal functions. Job restructuring may include transferring tasks to another employee, assigning different tasks to the person with a disability, and/or eliminating tasks that the person cannot perform. For example, a marginal function of an administrative assistant's position might involve answering telephones for thirty minutes each day. A person who is deaf would be unable to perform that function, thereby necessitating that it be reassigned to another employee. Job restructuring is an effective and usually inexpensive accommodation strategy, but it is limited to marginal or secondary functions of the position. Essential functions, which should be specified in written job descriptions, are not subject to restructuring.

Modification of Work Schedules

Modified work schedules offer a reasonable accommodation that is usually inexpensive and often easy to arrange. This option includes both flexible (working the same number of hours on a different schedule) and reduced time assignments. The effects of a disability may seem to necessitate significant changes in an employee's schedule, but slight modifications can often yield impressive results. For example, a person with multiple sclerosis who encounters chronic fatigue has difficulty sustaining her physical stamina in the afternoon. Rather than reducing her schedule to mornings only, she might request an extended two-hour lunch period during which she could take a nap and regain her strength for the afternoon. She might then work an extra hour at the end of her shift to make up the time.

Reassignment to Another Position

In some cases, an accommodation may not be possible for the employee's present position but would be feasible for another job. If the employer and employee agree that the other position would be more appropriate, they may consider reassignment to that position as an accommodation option. Importantly, reassignment may not be used to limit, segregate, or otherwise discriminate against the employee. The new position should be vacant at the time of reassignment or expected to be vacant within a reasonable time frame. If the employee is qualified for the new position, it should be at least equivalent in pay and status to the previous job. If the employee is not qualified for reassignment to an equal-status position, the employer may offer him a lower-grade position.

Modification of Equipment

Unless associated costs constitute an undue hardship for the employer, employees with disabilities must have access to the equipment that is routinely used on their jobs. Often, existing equipment can be modified with slight expense and minor inconvenience. The following are two MS-specific examples:

Problem: A secretary with MS experiences numbness in her hands and has difficulty turning a dictation machine on and off.

Solution: A foot pedal is installed to control the machine.

Problem: A computer programmer with a visual impairment resulting from MS finds it difficult to read the monitor at his work station.

Solution: His employer installs a software package that enlarges images on the screen.

Installation of New Equipment

When existing equipment cannot be modified, the employer must consider new equipment that will enable the employee to perform the essential functions of her job. The employer is only required, however, to provide equipment for that particular job, not equipment to be used outside of work in the employee's personal life. The following are two examples of new equipment accommodations:

Problem: A file clerk with MS-related tremors in his hands finds it difficult to access and manipulate files.

Solution: His employer installs a swiveling "lazy Susan" file cabinet to enable him to reach materials more easily.

Problem: A newspaper editor with MS has difficulty with the large volume of reading that is required on her job because of fatigue and a slight visual impairment.

Solution: Her employer purchases a closed-circuit magnification machine to reduce eye strain and increase her productivity.

Provision of Qualified Readers and Interpreters

Readers and interpreters are often provided as reasonable accommodations for people with visual and hearing impairments. Trained assistants facilitate access to written and spoken communication, and they can serve a valuable function in enabling people with disabilities to do their jobs. Although personal assistance of this kind can be expensive, most employees who use readers and interpreters need them for only a small portion of the day.

Modification of Application and Examination Procedures and Training Materials

Title I requires that application and examination procedures and training materials be made accessible to people with disabilities based on individual need. Applications and examinations must assess the ability, not the limitations, of the person to perform the essential functions of the position. If the application process requires an examination, the employer must give advance notice so that the applicant can request needed accommodations. Examination accommodations may include readers, scribes, extended time, a non-distractive environment, and/or elimination of items or sections that the examinee cannot complete due to disability.

If training or continuing education is offered, employers are required to make reasonable accommodations on an as-needed, as-requested basis. Training accommodations may include accessible sites, modified formats for materials (e.g., braille, large print, and simplified language), and modified administration of training (e.g., interpreters, readers, job coaches, and extended time).

Flexible Personal Leave Policies

Flexible personal leave is considered a reasonable accommodation when an employee requires time off due to her disability. Under that circumstance, the employer may allow her to use accrued leave, advance leave ("borrowing" from future accrued leave), and/or leave without pay. Flexible leave policies may be implemented to accommodate both the employee's disability and her responsibility for family members (spouse or dependent child) who have disabilities.

Table 5-1 presents additional examples of reasonable accommodations that are of interest to people with MS.

Table 5-1. Accommodation Strategies for People with Multiple Sclerosis

Job Function	MS Factor	Possible Accommodation
Entering place of business	Muscular weakness	Restructuring of existing facilities, e.g., electronic door opener
Supervising activities in the gymnasium (climbing and standing)	Loss of strength in lower extremities	Restructuring of the job, e.g. supervising study halls instead of activities in the gymnasium
Conducting medical examinations more than 8 hours a day	Fatigue	Modification of work schedules, e.g., 8-hour day with breaks
Supervising construction operations and activities	Fatigue and coordination/balance problems	Reassignment to another position, e.g., reassignment to sitting, indoor job as manager
Turning dictation machine off	Numbness of hands, problems with eye/hand coordination	Modification of equipment, e.g., installation of foot pedal to control equipment
Remembering details, setting priorities, and developing production schedules	Impact on cognitive skills and short-term memory	Installation of new equipment, e.g., portable computer with printer hook-up
Reading reports and self-generated typing	Blurred vision	Provision of qualified readers and interpreters, e.g., reader/proofer in office when needed

What Does "Undue Hardship" Mean?

"Undue hardship" refers to an accommodation that would be unduly costly, extensive, and/or disruptive. For example, does the accommodation cost more than alternatives that are equally effective in removing work limitations? Does it require extensive renovations that would disrupt the business? Would it affect other employees or customers in a negative way? If the answers are "yes," an employer is not required to provide the requested accommodation.

Undue hardship is decided on a case-by-case basis. Factors influencing whether an accommodation is considered an undue hardship on the employer include the size of the business and the availability of resources to reduce the net cost of the accommodation to the employer. An undue hardship for one business may not be an undue hardship for another. Don't limit your range of options by deciding in advance that a certain solution constitutes an undue hardship for your employer. The "win-win" approach will help you to explore a wide range of options with your employer.

Planning Your Approach

Now that you understand the key employment provisions of the ADA and your civil rights under them, the next step involves discussing your on-the-job needs with your employer. We believe that an informal and friendly dialogue between you and your employer without mentioning the ADA is the best way to start.

Before you say anything to your employer, you should do some homework. Analyze the problems you are having. This guide provides some suggestions about solutions. You might also want to call the nearest chapter of the National Multiple Sclerosis Society or your state's vocational rehabilitation office to learn about additional solutions that have worked for others. Generate a written list of accommodations and then analyze it carefully. Would any of these accommodations increase your productivity? Explore each accommodation strategy in terms of its potential effectiveness for you. Then consider it from your employer's standpoint. Would it be cost-effective? Does it alter the nature of the business? Now write your list a second time, putting the best suggestions first.

Next identify the appropriate person with whom you should meet. You may feel most comfortable speaking with your immediate supervisor, but company policy may require that you discuss these issues with someone in the personnel or human resources department. Some employers insist on a written communication. Find out what is required.

You now know to whom you will speak, and after reading the sections that follow you will know the points you should cover. However, most people find it difficult to discuss their MS with their employers. In effect, you are informing your employer that you are no longer able to do your job without accommodations. Rehearse your presentation with a friend or advisor so that you have the best possible chance for success. Remember to stress the experience you have gained as an employee of the business. Employers do not want to lose seasoned and loyal workers. Replacing an experienced employee costs time and money, and it always involves an element of risk for an employer.

Discussing the Request with Your Employer

Here are some tips on preparing for your meeting:

1. Dress in work-appropriate clothes. Wear what you would normally wear to work.

2. Arrive on time.

3. Thank your employer for meeting with you. Then begin by introducing the purpose of the meeting.

4. Use appropriate body language. Maintain eye contact during the conversation, squarely face your employer, lean slightly forward, nod to indicate attention, and assume a receptive facial expression.

5. Use appropriate verbal language. Answer questions honestly and directly. Use nonadversarial terms: "I would like to explore with you . . .," "It makes sense for both of us to . . . ," and "Together, we could come up with . . . ." Avoid saying "I want . . . ," "I'm entitled to . . . ," or "You have to. . . ."

6. Be positive. Focus on ways that your enhanced productivity will benefit your employer. Don't dwell on the past, and don't react angrily to resistance.

The ADA clearly states that you should be involved in deciding what specific accommodations your employer should implement. The collaboration phase of the "win-win" process involves you and your employer working together to identify the accommodations that would benefit both of you. As you follow these guidelines, keep in mind the mutual benefit of effective on-the-job accommodations.

Remember that although the ADA requires that your employer provide a reasonable accommodation, the employer does not have to provide the most reasonable one from your point of view. It is important to be willing to compromise.

1. Give your employer a copy of the list you generated at home, with accommodations ranked in order of your preference. Ask your employer to rank them in order of his or her preference, as a way to start the process.

2. Compare the two lists. If you and your employer do not agree, point out again the mutual benefits of the accommodation you prefer. Attempt to convince your employer that your idea is the right one, rather than pointing out that he or she is wrong.

3. Be prepared to negotiate an agreement. You can negotiate from a position of strength by keeping in mind your ADA protections. It may not be necessary to state your right to appeal your employer's decision, but remember that it does exist.

4. If you reach an agreement, be sure to discuss follow-up procedures and agree on a timetable for action. If your employer proposes an unreasonable compromise, ask for time to think it over. If you cannot agree, suggest that you both think about it some more. In either case, schedule another meeting within ten days.

Resources: Who Can Help?

As you and your employer work together to identify and implement reasonable accommodations that meet the needs of both parties, it may be helpful to call on outside resources for consultation (Rumrill, Roessler, & Reed, 1995). Two important national networks are ABLEDATA and the Job Accommodation Network. ABLEDATA is located in Silver Spring, Maryland (8455 Colesville Road, Suite 935, 20910-3319; 800-227-0216) and provides specific information on technological devices including functions, costs, and vendors. Housed at West Virginia University in Morgantown, JAN consults with private industry and individuals concerning job accommodations and technology (800-526-7234) and the ADA (800-232-9675).

In addition to these excellent accommodation resources, you can benefit from the legal assistance of several government agencies. The U.S. Equal Employment Opportunity Commission (EEOC, 1801 L Street, NW, Washington, DC 20507; 800-669-EEOC [voice], 800-800-3302 [TDD]) enforces Title I provisions and offers information, referrals to other sources, and technical assistance regarding Title I. The U.S. Department of Justice, Civil Rights Division (P.O. Box 66118, Washington, DC 20035-6118; 202-514-0301 [voice], 202-514-0381 [TDD]) enforces Titles II (Public Services) and III (Public Accommodations) of the ADA. The Internal Revenue Service (1111 Constitution Avenue, NW, Washington, DC 20224; 800-829-3676 [voice], 800-829-4059 [TDD] provides information regarding tax credits, exemptions, and deductions associated with hiring and accommodating qualified employees with disabilities.

Another valuable resource for people with MS, rehabilitation professionals, and employers alike is the National Multiple Sclerosis Society (733 Third Avenue, New York, NY 10017; 212-986-3240). Appendix B presents a directory of the Society's local chapters. See also Chapter 7.

The accommodation process can be somewhat complicated, but help is available! Before you move to the implementation phase, there are a few more resources you may wish to consider (see Appendix C; Equal Employment Opportunity Commission, 1992).

Implementing Reasonable Accommodations

In most cases, you and your employer will identify a mutually acceptable accommodation plan. Because the course of MS is unpredictable, you must monitor the effectiveness of your on-the-job accommodations and communicate frequently with your employer. Here are a few other points to remember:

1. Take some time to become familiar with your accommodation. If the accommodation involves technology, ask for appropriate training.

2. Be aware of changes in your medical condition and how those changes might be addressed through the "win-win" process. Remember that the ADA does not limit the number or types of accommodations that can be provided. You may need to ask for one again later on.

3. Keep your employer informed about your condition, how your accommodations work, and your general job performance. Your employer will appreciate updates on your progress, and you will both enjoy the benefits of a good working relationship.

But What If?

If the collaborative "win-win" strategy does not result in acceptable solutions to your needs, if you see signs of discriminatory conduct on your employer's part, or if you believe that the accommodation he or she has chosen would not enable you to do your job, you have legal recourse.

The ADA requires your employer to respond to your request in a timely manner. If your employer does not respond within ten working days, make a follow-up telephone call or personal contact to arrange a meeting. If you cannot negotiate a satisfactory solution with your employer, you have the right to appeal outcomes of the "win-win" approach. Bring in the ADA if, and only if, the collaborative process breaks down and your employer is unwilling to participate any further. You may choose to file a formal complaint with the Equal Employment Opportunity Commission (EEOC). You can find this number in your local telephone directory under the United States Government heading.

Do not delay in making contact with the EEOC if you experience problems. A charge of discrimination must be filed with the EEOC within one hundred eighty days (about six months) from the time of the alleged discriminatory act. You may also want to secure the help of a disability rights advocate or attorney.

For more information on legal or advocacy help, contact the nearest National Multiple Sclerosis Society Chapter (see Appendix B), your state or local bar associations, state or local advocates for people with disabilities, and other voluntary health agencies or client assistance projects in your area. Do not assume legal help will be too expensive for you without investigating these resources.

We hope that the "win-win" strategy will work for you, but if it does not, you have rights under the ADA. The EEOC, disability advocates, and attorneys are available to help you protect your rights.

Conclusion

The "win-win" approach is designed to assist you in collaborating with your employer to identify and implement solutions to your on-the-job needs. Mutually beneficial and cost-effective steps for maintaining your productivity on the job are the ultimate goals. By identifying your needs, understanding your legal rights under the ADA, and keeping in mind cooperative negotiation strategies for discussing accommodations with your employer, you have prepared yourself to be a confident and effective "win-win" strategist.

Summary

Title I of the ADA provides specific employment protections for people with MS and other disabilities, but it requires the applicant or employee to play an active part in identifying her needs, communicating with her employer, and initiating remedies in the event of discrimination. On a general level, people with MS need to know that the ADA:

1. Provides civil rights protection for people with disabilities in broad areas of social activity, including employment.

2. Prohibits employment discrimination on the basis of disability.

3. Requires most public and private employers to provide reasonable accommodations that allow qualified people with disabilities to perform essential job functions.

4. Prevents employers from asking disability-related questions on application forms or at job interviews.

5. Requires the applicant or employee to disclose his or her disability before becoming eligible for reasonable accommodations.

6. Requires employers and employees to work together in identifying and implementing accommodations.

7. Provides specific legal remedies for people who have been discriminated against.

Specifically, people with MS need to know the ways in which the illness could hinder their job performance. They also need information concerning solutions, or reasonable accommodations, that could help them overcome those limitations. Fortunately, there are many excellent resources that can assist in every aspect of the accommodation process. Perhaps most importantly, people with MS and other disabilities need to develop and practice strategies for communicating their needs to employers that are both nonadversarial and compatible with the provisions of Title I of the ADA. In closing, readers are reminded that reasonable accommodations are, indeed, a matter of civil rights, but the best reason for their implementation from the employer's perspective is that they (1) are cost-effective, (2) enhance the employee's productivity, and (3) enable the business or agency to retain qualified and capable workers.

Chapter 6

Tax Benefits and Work Incentives

Steven B. Mendelsohn

The tax law includes a number of provisions that can be of great benefit to people with multiple sclerosis or other chronic conditions. Through credits, deductions, or other mechanisms, these provisions provide favorable tax treatment for a variety of costs incurred as the results of working, obtaining technology and training, the purchase of services needed to live independently at home, and in general to secure and maintain the best possible quality of life.

People with multiple sclerosis or other adult-onset disabilities frequently face curtailment of their work in the prime of their careers and as they are approaching the height of their earning potential. Coming almost out of nowhere, as it frequently does, and with no warning or reason to expect it, the diagnosis can itself be a profoundly disruptive event. It can shatter expectations and plans, create personal and family stress, and, perhaps worst of all, give rise to prolonged and profound uncertainty and doubt as to what the future may hold.

While recent developments in medical and pharmacologic research hold significant new hope for many people, the course of MS remains unpredictable. No one knows exactly how and over what time frame it will affect a variety of functional capabilities in each individual. However, it is predictable that some functional limitations may occur in mobility, vision, stamina, or other areas.

Faced with the economic impact of MS, it is vital to remember that alternative strategies frequently exist for sustaining economic productivity. With the development of assistive technology and the passage of the Americans with Disabilities Act (ADA), there is growing recognition that disability need not obstruct productivity and achievement. The prospects for continued work and employment for people with MS are greater than ever before. But the assistive technology, attendant services, and reasonable accommodations often required to make this possible are not free. How much they cost and who will pay for them are key issues.

If you use a wheelchair, your ability to work may hinge on workplace accessibility. If your vision is impaired, print enlargement, synthetic speech computer output, or other technologies may be the margin of difference between being able and being unable to continue working at an appropriate level of function. Flexible work hours or the opportunity to work at home may be the key for those who experience fatigue. For those who can no longer drive or lift, the services of an assistant may prove instrumental.

Legal provisions have helped to create opportunities to effectively implement technology for employment and work. Title I of the ADA, as well as other federal and state laws, requires employers to provide reasonable accommodations where appropriate, including technology. The scope and applicability of such antidiscrimination and equal opportunity laws is beyond the subject of this chapter. Our focus here is on the tax law provisions that can help to subsidize the add-on costs of working in the presence of MS, and on other work incentives in federal law that can further contribute to this goal.

The Internal Revenue Code contains important incentives, both for businesses to provide accommodations and for individuals who must meet some or all of their work-related and accommodations costs. Tax subsidization of an expenditure does not, of course, generate the cash flow necessary to pay the cost in question and will not be meaningful to all businesses. Such subsidization is likely to be of little value to those that are too small or too unprofitable to owe any taxes at the end of the year. The existence of major tax benefits for accommodating working people with disabilities is likely to make no difference to employers in the nonprofit or governmental sectors, who pay no taxes. Individuals will also differ in their opportunity to benefit, depending on their income levels, overall tax profiles, and ability to anticipate and plan for needed expenditures. Nevertheless, even those who cannot obtain the full benefit of the law can often gain *some* advantage from it. This advantage, large or small, should be known to all who stand to gain from utilizing what the law offers.

Miscellaneous Itemized Deductions and Impairment-Related Work Expenses

Most of the costs people incur in performing their jobs qualify for tax deductibility under the Miscellaneous Itemized Deductions (MIDs) of section 67(b) of the Internal Revenue Code. However, there are important limitations on the range of employment expenses that will be eligible for this deduction. MIDs, including unreimbursed employee business expenses, are deductible only to the extent that they exceed two percent of your adjusted gross income (AGI). Moreover, many expenses incurred by people with disabilities do not fall within the traditional profile of employee business expenses, and are therefore likely to become issues in tax audits. This includes expenses such as those for attendant services or for technology that can be used both in and out of work.

Working people with disabilities therefore need to know about the related itemized deduction category known as impairment-related work expenses (IRWEs), added to the Code in 1986 as Section 67(d). The provision assists people with disabilities in two important ways:

▲ It exempts IRWEs from the two percent threshold applicable to other work expenses. For those who can itemize, this means that their entire IRWE costs are deductible, not merely those that exceed the two percent of AGI threshold.

▲ The provision defines IRWEs in a manner that eliminates much of the confusion between personal and employment expenses that might otherwise exist.

The law defines IRWEs as: "expenses of a handicapped individual . . . for attendant care services at the individual's place of employment and other expenses in connection with such place of employment that are necessary for such individual to be able to work. . . ." While the law includes no reference to assistive technology (AT), such equipment does clearly fall within the "other" costs category. Likewise, the law does not require any particular diagnosis or medical certification, only that the individual meet a standard that is phrased in terms of functional limitations that constitute or result in limitations of one or more major life activities. Moving, walking, seeing, remembering, and other functional limitations commonly experienced in MS would readily come within this definition (see also IRC Sec. 190).

As this definition suggests, three elements must be present for an expenditure to qualify as an IRWE:

▲ The expense must be incurred to enable the individual to work;

▲ It must be made by an individual who meets the definition of "handicapped"; and

▲ It must be of a nature that would not be necessary in the absence of the disability or functional limitation in question.

These elements seem straightforward. Even necessity, which is perhaps the most difficult of them, is not construed to mean that the individual could not work or would be fired but for the goods or services in question.

Some concern has arisen over the episodic nature of multiple sclerosis. Accommodation needs may change as exacerbations and remissions occur. A given item of work-related technology may be needed at one time but not at another. This does not jeopardize its eligibility to be claimed as an IRWE. The status of the technology as an IRWE would properly be called into question only if it were used on a routine basis when not needed to help overcome the functional limitations of the disability, or if it were used "other than incidentally" for personal, non-work-related activities.

Does this mean that someone who acquired a computer because of difficulty in handwriting would have to cease using it during periods of remission? Such a question has never been addressed by the IRS regulations or in tax law cases, but the answer would appear to be "no." Permanent recovery or long-term suppression of symptoms aside, the purpose for having the technology remains that of overcoming the functional limitations of the disability, and future exacerbations are likely.

Some distinction might be in order between the basic computer and its specialized software or adaptive peripherals, such as a modified keyboard or an enlarging screen. Although the prospects are remote, you might be called upon to prove that the base computer would not have been acquired and used but for the disability; however, this motivation would be self-evident in the case of such disability-related add-ons. Still, the computer itself would routinely qualify as an MID (if IRWE designation presented a problem) if it was not paid for by the employer but was used in the workplace.

Many people with MS find it preferable to work at home. Given the general growth in telecommuting, such opportunities appear somewhat more prevalent than they were in the past. A person who works at home may do so either as the operator of a home-based business or as an employee. In either case, most of their disability-related equipment and services costs should qualify for deductibility. The specific circumstances of the work will determine the appropriate tax law categories to be used. If you are employed, the employee business expense and IRWE provisions should continue to apply, subject to two limitations discussed in the next paragraph. If you are self-employed, either as an entrepreneur or as an independent contractor, your accommodation expenses should be treated like any other costs of operating the business and should normally be deductible on Schedule C (Profit or Loss from Self-Employment) or on the equivalent forms used for determining the taxable income from a partnership or corporation.

There are two limitations on the applicability of the MID and IRWE provisions for work performed at home. One derives from the ambiguity surrounding the words "at" or "in connection with" in the IRWE statute. Although definitive interpretation by regulations or by the courts is still awaited, indications from the nonbinding examples given in a number of IRS informational publications over the years suggest that location would not preclude deductibility, at least in those instances in which the personal and nonpersonal components of the goods or services could be easily separated. For example, the use of a reader's services during periods of visual limitation would be all right, as long as one could separate time spent on work-related activities from time spent reading other things.

What about such services as those of an attendant who assists you in getting up and ready for work in the morning? Such services would not qualify as MIDs because they are deemed inherently personal in nature. Additionally, they might well be better deducted as medical care expenses. Would they qualify as IRWEs for the employed person? The answer remains uncertain. On the one hand, it could be argued that such services are not work-related since you would need them even if you were not going to work. On the other hand, the time spent preparing for work can be distinguished from that spent getting ready to spend the day in other pursuits. Again, even if the IRWE deduction is available, taxpayers may wish to utilize the medical expense deduction, although there is a practical limitation in that medical expenses are deductible only to the extent that they exceed 7.5 percent of the year's AGI.

The second major limitation on tax deductibility of home-based work-related or business expenses is more troubling. It arises from the concept of "listed property" (IRC Sec. 280f). There are limitations in the deductibility of computers (but not adaptive peripherals), automobiles, cellular phones, and other devices, which everyone is presumed to want (and which Congress and the IRS assume everyone will try to justify as a business expense if they can). To qualify as employee business expenses, items of listed property must be specifically "for the convenience" of the employer, or they must be required by the employer as a condition of employment. The listed property issue poses a slightly different problem for home-based businesses. The way in which the equipment can be deducted in terms of the number of years over which its cost must be allocated depends on the ability to document that its use is solely for business.

People who work at home, either as employees or as entrepreneurs, have long assumed their entitlement to a home office deduction. In the past, this deduction has been based on the proportion of the space and of utility, mortgage or rent, or other costs that can be applied to their work space. However, the home office deduction has not been automatic since the Supreme Court's 1993 Soliman decision. Not only must one work at home, but the home office must actually be the individual's principal place of business. An anesthesiologist who used his home office to prepare bills and reports, keep and maintain records, and so forth was denied a deduction for the office because the business of an anesthesiologist is conducted in a hospital, not in an office. He did not see patients, prepare syringes, or perform the other activities of his work at home. Contrary to popular opinion, preparing bills was not deemed a central element of a physician's work.

The Medical Expense Deduction

Apropos health care, it is important to remember that the medical expense deduction can also play a role in facilitating the technology that may be needed in order to work. This itemized deduction (see IRC Sec. 213) is broader in scope than is commonly realized. It applies to most physicians' services in diagnosis and treatment (except for certain cosmetic surgeries) and to prescription drugs, but it is also available to help defray the costs of much more. The law allows the deduction for anything that affects a "structure or function" of the body. To the extent that much AT does this, and results in some degree of mitigation (even if not in traditional clinical terms), the medical expense deduction has been granted for a wide variety of equipment and devices. These include telecommunications devices for the deaf (TDDs), closed-caption TV decoders, braille writing equipment, and, of course, wheelchairs, canes, walkers, van lifts, and adaptive driving controls. [Cases and rulings on these deductions are collected and analyzed in *Tax Options and Strategies for People with Disabilities*, 2nd edition, by Steven B. Mendelsohn (New York: Demos Vermande, 1996, Chapter 4.]

Beyond representing a fall-back strategy for subsidizing the costs of work-related technology, the medical expense deduction may in some instances actually represent the most effective approach to achieving this goal because not all work-related items are used *solely* for work. A powered wheelchair, a lift-equipped van, or other devices may be indispensable for getting to and from or for performing one's job, but their use may not be limited to the vocational setting. For that reason, they may not qualify for the IRWE deduction. Also, items ranging from canes to eyeglasses to service dogs are deemed "inherently personal" in nature, even if they are used primarily in a work setting and therefore deductible only as health care items.

In contrast, nothing in the law deprives an otherwise deductible medical care expense of its favored tax treatment simply because it is partly used in work-related pursuits. There was a time when equipment such as a van lift would have been deductible as a medical expense only if it were used for the sole purpose of facilitating trips to and from medical care. Happily, that time has passed, as has the era when what are considered to be capital expenses (expenses for the acquisition of durable equipment or property expected to last more than one year and not to be consumed by repeated use as supplies) were often denied medical expense deduction status.

Because the medical expense deduction is limited to those eligible costs that exceed 7.5 percent of AGI, some portion of your unreimbursed medical expenses will always be lost to you as far as the deduction is concerned. For this reason, tax planning can be especially useful in maximizing the value of this deduction. Use of the medical expense category for AT should be considered if your other medical expenses have already reached the 7.5 percent threshold. Additionally, to the extent that your medical costs can often be anticipated, such as those for AT devices, efforts should be made to group as many of your health expenses as possible in a single year, especially when this will bring total health care costs over the 7.5 percent mark. Remember that medical expenses must be deducted in the year in which they are incurred. Items purchased with credit cards (although not necessarily with other kinds of loans) are deemed paid for when the credit card charge is made. It does not matter how long you take to pay off the bank or other card company (see Revenue Ruling 78-39).

For those who work at home, the medical expense deduction can also help to reduce the costs of home modifications necessary to accommodate a disability. Such home modification expenses are eligible for the medical expense deduction if they are required to enable you to continue living in your home, to assure your safety, to facilitate your movement and access, or to permit you to engage in activities of daily living such as getting to the bathroom, the kitchen, or your bed. Your allowable deduction may be less than the full cost of the modifications, however, because they are deductible only to the degree that they do not increase the value of the property. Any increase in value, typically as determined by an appraisal, will be subtracted from the available deduction. If, for example, your home modifications cost $10,000 but increased the value of the property by $2,000, the maximum deduction available to you would be $8,000. The IRS publishes a list of modifications that it considers as having no impact on property values, but most routine home modifications of the kind that people with MS frequently make do not increase the value of their homes. So far as the use of the medical expense deduction to subsidize necessary modifications to your home is involved, it should make no difference that you also use part of it for business or work purposes.

Although both business and medical deductions can be used to help defray the costs of AT, never assume that these two deduction categories are interchangeable. The medical expense deduction is broader as far as the context of device use is concerned, serving as it does to cover devices used partly in work as well as in personal living, but there are major limitations on what devices qualify for the deduction. For that deduction to be available, you must be able to show a connection between the expenditure and the mitigation of a health problem or of the functional limitations associated with a disability. The case for medical deductibility is most easily made with devices that are designed or modified specifically for use in the context of a disability and for services that no one would want or need but for the presence of a disability. For instance, a one-handed keyboard for a computer is of no use to someone who has ordinary motor function, so would easily be understood as mitigating the limitation in mobility. However, the computer to which that keyboard attaches is quite another matter. It can be difficult for a taxpayer to prove that he would not have bought a computer save for the disability and to show that it meets disability-related needs as distinguished from the normal range of needs for which people purchase computers.

People with multiple sclerosis often incur work-related costs for vocational rehabilitation or for skills retraining needed to develop new methods of doing their former work or in order to engage in new vocational pursuits. People who incur educational or training costs in order to improve performance in their current jobs usually are entitled to deduct these costs as MIDs. The MID category would also apply to in-service or job-retention and enhancement training needed by a person with MS. Someone in this situation must also consider whether the IRWE deduction could apply. Its cost should qualify as an IRWE if training is specifically related to the disability, as in the use of AT that will be used in the office. The distinction between MIDs and IRWEs may not matter if your MIDs already exceed two percent of your AGI for the year. You can simply add the AT training expenses to your other MIDs without losing any tax benefit.

The situation is more complex when it relates to retraining for *new* work. Enlightened medical or disability insurers should fund such training and recognize that it is cost-effective when compared with a prolonged period of economic dependency. However, such a response is not yet common. One would likewise wish that the vocational rehabilitation (VR) system operated by state rehabilitation agencies under the Federal Rehabilitation Act would contribute, but here again there are often problems.

The individual who must contribute to the cost of such rehabilitation or retraining expenses must deal with the problem that training or educational expenses incurred in search of a new job are not ordinarily deductible. Job search expenses as such can be, but not the training involved in preparing for some new line of work. This limitation can be a significant injustice for people obliged by disability to enter a new line of work as an alternative to dependency. One partial solution may be to investigate whether any of the training might qualify for the medical expense deduction. To the extent that the training is provided by those whose orientation and qualifications are related to the restoration of function, including adaptive strategies for performing various tasks, it may be permissible to characterize some of these general rehabilitative costs as medical in nature; this would include the services of professionals such as physical or occupational therapists or low vision specialists. Training that is specifically applicable to a particular vocation, or to vocational as distinguished from broader living skills, could not be so characterized, but the potential of this approach for much of the basic rehabilitation service that people may need should be discussed at length with a knowledgeable tax adviser.

The reference to a "knowledgeable tax adviser" brings us to yet another major issue. Many accountants, tax planners, and tax preparers know little about disability-related issues and deductions. Indeed, why should they be expected to know more than others in the general society? This can be a serious problem for taxpayers with disabilities or for families with a member who has a disability. However competent and skillful, most tax professionals are not intimately familiar with those obscure provisions of the law that are of greatest concern to people with disabilities. Even if familiar with the law, they are not likely to possess the factual information about the disability to know how the law applies. Finally, unless the matter is brought to the attention of the accountant or other expert, you may never discuss such things as the presence of a person with a disability in the family tax equation, the fact that some equipment purchased may have been assistive technology, or the need to plan for meeting disability-related costs. Even if these issues are mentioned, the potential for discomfort, unstated assumptions, or other harmful emotional reactions cannot be discounted. A tax adviser cannot do an optimal job if she is inhibited in asking the necessary questions and gathering the necessary data, no matter how qualified or well-intentioned.

Incentives for Businesses

Thus far I have discussed tax benefits for individuals who must finance some or all of their own accommodations. But the law does more. Many people believe that its role in facilitating the public policy of inclusion falls far short of what might be expected and hoped for. Although outside the scope of this chapter, there are many respects in which tax law fails to structure its incentives and disincentives in a manner that is fully consistent with current public policy. The debate over the proper role of the tax system in this area is increasingly complicated by the growing belief that the tax system should not be used as a social policy instrument. But let us make no mistake. There is no conceivable tax system or structure that is without impact on social conditions in our country. Every tax proposal embodies a social agenda. The only real difference between those who advocate an income tax and those who favor a consumption tax, between those who favor a flat tax and those who support a graduated income tax, is that some are more candid than others regarding the social goals that lie behind the economic statistics and models they cite.

There are three major incentives in current law for businesses to hire and accommodate people with multiple sclerosis or other disabilities. The first is nonspecific but important nonetheless. Businesses are accorded deductibility for the "ordinary and necessary" expenses incurred in their operation. They are given considerable latitude to determine what costs they must incur. With a few exceptions such as excessive compensation to owners or key officials and others not pertinent to this discussion, their discretion will suffice to cover the costs of AT or other accommodations, just as it covers the costs of routine technology provided for the use of other employees. Businesses asked to provide AT frequently overlook this fact. Equally important, they often apply the wrong accounting techniques to determine what the AT will cost. In conversations with executives and accountants, I have often noted a tendency to ask what the entire cost of technology or other accommodations for an employee with a disability would be. The better question would be to ask the amount by which accommodating an employee with a disability would exceed the cost of hiring someone else. Ideally, this calculation should be done on the basis of long-term budget forecasts, including anticipated equipment life cycles and replacement schedules.

Additionally, some business incentives are targeted specifically to people with disabilities, such as the architectural and transportation barriers removal deduction (ATB) for the "handicapped and elderly." Normally when a firm spends money to renovate or modify facilities or vehicles, it treats such costs as capital expenses, which simply means that they are not entirely deductible in the year they are incurred but must be depreciated (spread out) over a number of years. The ATB allows some of these costs to be recategorized as ordinary or operating expenses, making them fully deductible in the year in which the money was spent, up to a $15,000 annual limit. The law does not create a new deduction, but it greatly accelerates the rate at which the benefit can be accrued.

The ATB is available to businesses of any size. However, its use is complicated. The regulations (IRS Regs. Secs. 1.190-1 et seq.) create very detailed requirements concerning what constitutes a qualifying barrier removal expense. A firm that reduces the steep slope of an entryway, widens a doorway, or makes the bathrooms accessible must do so according to specific design standards. Most people who know about the ATB deduction think of it as applicable to the area of public accommodations, as a way that businesses can make their premises and facilities more accessible to disabled customers or other members of the public. The provision can indeed serve this role, but it also has great value in accommodating employees and job applicants.

The third incentive worthy of discussion here is the disabled access credit (DAC) (IRC Sec. 44). Enacted shortly after the passage of the ADA in 1990, this credit was intended to insulate small businesses from possible economic hardship associated with compliance with the Act. In a sense, the provision is redundant, since the ADA itself provides that "undue hardship" or "undue burden" shall be available as defenses to compliance requests that would be too costly or difficult. Nevertheless, the credit provides incentives to compliance and reduces the number of cases in which a request is likely to give rise to a valid undue burden claim.

Unlike the barrier removal deduction, the disabled access credit applies only to small businesses, but the term *small business* is liberally defined. For purposes of the DAC, a small business is defined as one with thirty or fewer full-time employees, or one with gross receipts for the preceding year of under $1 million. The law allows businesses that meet either of these standards a fifty percent tax credit, for up to $10,000 per year after an initial $250 exclusion, for what are termed *eligible access expenditures*. Again, most such expenditures would normally qualify for deduction as ordinary and necessary business expenses. The availability of the credit makes them much more valuable, since a credit comes directly off your tax bill while a deduction simply lowers taxable income. A firm that incurred $10,250 in eligible access expenses would be entitled to reduce its tax bill for the year by $5,000.

There are major limitations on the use of the credit for structural modifications to buildings or facilities, but it is exceptionally useful in meeting other accommodation and access expenses. These include the acquisition or modification of equipment; the provision of readers, interpreters, or other effective methods of communication; the removal of communications barriers; and the provision of "auxiliary aids and services."

Here too, although commonly thought of as a public accommodations measure, the credit can be used to facilitate the access of employees and would-be employees. As with the ATB, there is no requirement that a specific individual be identified as benefiting from the access expenditures before they are made. This, of course, does not preclude the needs of a particular individual from stimulating such efforts.

Because the DAC applies to small businesses, concerns may arise that some firms will have too little income to benefit fully from the credit the law makes available. However, even if a company's income for the year is insufficient to fully utilize its available credit, a remarkable feature of the law prevents its unused value from being forfeited. The unused portion of the credit can still be available in other years. This is so because the DAC is one of a number of credits comprising what is called the "general business credit" (IRC Sec. 38). Available income does serve as a limitation on the use of these credits, and there are some other limitations as well. But "carry-over" is available when a disabled access or other general business credit cannot be fully absorbed in the year in which the expense was incurred. The unused credit can be carried back for up to three years or forward for up to a full fifteen years. With such flexibility, it is likely that all but the most short-lived of firms will be able to obtain the full value of the credit that is available to them.

As indicated earlier, expenses can qualify for the ATB or the DAC when undertaken proactively—before identifying a particular individual who will benefit. Nevertheless, those who are intended to benefit must meet requirements of the law. In the case of the disabled access credit, eligible access expenditures must be designed to facilitate access for those people who meet the ADA's definition of disability. The applicability of the ADA hinges on the existence of a physical or mental impairment that "substantially limits one or more major life activities." Barrier removal expenses will only qualify if they are incurred to remove barriers to those who meet the statute's definition of "handicapped" or "elderly," as set forth previously.

The DAC and the ATB can apply to the businesses of people with disabilities who are self-employed. Although someone who owns or controls the finances of a small business should avoid using the firm's funds to meet personal expenses, the law allows a small business such as a sole proprietorship to meet the legitimate disability-related costs of its operation, as well as its other ordinary and necessary costs.

A home-based business that needs to accommodate customers, clients, or patients with disabilities should also be able to avail itself of these provisions of the Internal Revenue Code. Problems will arise if expenditures affect parts of the house used only for personal living. However, if there is only one doorway to the building, the installation of a ramp to accommodate wheelchair access will not fail to qualify for tax-favored treatment simply because both the residents and customers are able to use it.

The high degree of unpredictability in the course of MS raises legal as well as practical questions, and has implications for the application of the tax law to the situations faced by people with MS. At times, many individuals with MS can function much as they did prior to the onset of the disease. At other times, mobility, vision, fatigue, or other problems may arise, abate, and then recur in similar or different forms.

Insofar as many tax law provisions define disability in medical terms, such fluctuating conditions present several complex problems. People with MS need to understand which provisions of the law are linked to medical disability and what they offer in the way of tax benefits and opportunities for subsidization of disability-related expenses.

The answers to these questions depend on the particular tax law provision in question. We have already seen that fluctuations in functional capabilities should not ordinarily have a significant legal impact with such major work incentive provisions as the IRWE, the ATB and the DAC. However, if one is in remission at the time of the audit, some measure of skepticism from an unsophisticated tax examiner may be expected. Remission will likewise not endanger the deductibility of AT devices as medical expense deductions, but it could limit the deductibility of attendant services costs during the period of time when those services were not specifically required.

In general, an analysis of the issues will be helped by remembering how easy it is for those with little knowledge of conditions such as MS to confuse periods of remission with medical recovery. The fact that an item of equipment becomes temporarily unnecessary should not have an adverse impact on the deductibility of its costs, given the clinical picture, the likelihood of future use, and the motivation for incurring the expenses. After all, the deductibility of diabetic supplies is not jeopardized by an individual's ability to sufficiently control blood sugar through diet that he does not need insulin for some period of time.

The Child and Dependent Care Credit (IRC Sec. 21) may be important to those who must pay for the care of family members in order to work. This credit is available for the care of children under the age of thirteen or other disabled dependents, including spouses, who meet the law's definition of being "incapable of self-care." It has a maximum of $720 a year, or $1,440 for two or more care recipients.

The key point with multiple sclerosis may be that the determination of incapacity can in many cases be made on a daily basis. The approach used to compute the amount of the credit involves calculating the number of months of the year and the number of days in each month to which the credit is applicable. So far as capacity for self-care is concerned, this approach lends itself to the situations faced by people with fluctuating conditions.

Medical information can sometimes be helpful when a problem arises that relates to an individual's degree of incapacity. However, eligibility for the credit is not predicated on the findings or assertions of a physician. There are other instances in the

Internal Revenue Code in which the role of the doctor is far more central, where the physician in effect serves, willingly or otherwise, as gatekeeper for the tax system.

The Credit for the Elderly and the Permanently and Totally Disabled (CPT, as we shall call it) and the retirement funds' early withdrawal penalty waiver illustrate physician-mediated provisions. Let's take a closer look at these provisions and how they apply to conditions such as multiple sclerosis.

The CPT (IRC Sec.22) is important for low-income people who are over the age of sixty-five or for people under age sixty-five who have retired from work because of a "permanent and total disability." The role of a provision such as the CPT is quite different from the direct and indirect work incentive provisions discussed thus far. Those provisions were intended to subsidize or facilitate economic activity, but the CPT is aimed at mitigating some small part of the economic loss associated with the inability to work. Because its operation is triggered by such inability, it is not surprising that rigorous standards of diagnosis and medical evidence should be used. One cannot claim the credit unless a physician has certified the existence, nature, and severity of a condition that prevents an individual from working, is expected to either be of a long-term or definite duration, or is expected to result in death. Whether the disability needs to be periodically recertified by the physician depends on its nature.

A similar role is accorded to medical evidence and certification in connection with the provision allowing the waiver of penalties on the premature withdrawal of retirement funds (IRC Sec. 72). For those who withdraw funds early, typically before age fifty-nine and a half, a penalty tax or additional tax is assessed. It typically amounts to ten percent of the prematurely withdrawn amount.

The law permits exemption from the penalty when the withdrawal is made because a "permanent and total disability" that precipitated the early retirement. The penalty waiver does not depend on the precise use made of the withdrawn funds. Funds need not be spent directly for disability-related expenses, although they frequently are.

The definition of permanent and total disability in this context is essentially identical to that employed for the CPT. The test is incapacity to engage in "substantial gainful activity" due to a condition that can be expected to result in death or to continue for a long and indefinite period.

As with the CPT, the physician is the primary gatekeeper. The individual with MS may face the situation of meeting these definitions at certain times and not meeting them at others. In connection with retirement funds, for example, would the waiver be retroactively canceled and would the penalty after all have to be paid if a subsequent remission permitted return to work for some period of time? There have been a few cases in which subsequent return to work was held to invalidate the penalty waiver, but they appear to have involved situations in which the individual was never actually disabled and never really unable to work.

The best interpretation is that if an individual's diagnosis, prognosis, and dysfunctional level meet the statutory requirements at the time the funds are withdrawn, the subsequent periods of remission will not invalidate the tax benefit. Much to be considered here depends on level of income. If the subsequent ability to work results in regular, long-term economic activity that generates income comparable to what the individual was earning prior to the onset of the condition that resulted in premature withdrawal, there might well be a problem if the statute of limitations for auditing a prior return had not expired.

Another issue concerns blindness. People who meet the definition of legal blindness are entitled to an additional standard deduction. A person who may literally be legally blind on one day but not a week later must therefore ask when the diagnosis should be made. Strictly speaking, the last day of what we call the "taxable year" (for almost all individuals, December 31) is the key date. Much depends on the physician's assessment and write-up.

Fluctuating conditions present many challenges to the planning and living of daily life. Tax complications should not be among them. With this introduction to the issue, we hope that they can be dealt with more easily.

Other Work Incentives

Beyond tax law provisions such as those discussed previously, federal law also provides a number of other work incentives that may prove valuable to people with MS. Despite the disincentives that exist in various federal programs, the barriers that exist to efforts to return to work can be significantly reduced by knowledge of the work incentive provisions.

From taxes to social security, the fundamental problem throughout our legal code is the concept of ability or inability to work. People are classified as falling on one side of the line—they are entitled to benefits if they cannot work and not entitled to anything if they can. This division is far too simplistic for our present society. Advances in technology, developments in the management of progressive disease, changes in attitudes and expectations surrounding disability, and changes in the nature and organization of work in our society all contribute to the blurring of these convenient distinctions.

In broad terms there are two types of work incentive:

▲ Those such as vocational rehabilitation or veterans' training that involve the use of governmental funds to assist people in getting jobs; and

▲ Those such as the Social Security Act provisions that allow people with disabilities to become employed without losing all of their benefits (including insurance) until their ability to remain employed has been established and stabilized.

Most notable among such work incentive provisions are the trial work period (TWP) and the substantial gainful activity (SGA) concepts, which operate under the Social Security Disability Insurance (SSDI) program. Apart from being covered under the social security program, the test for eligibility under SSDI is that of having a "medically determinable illness or disability" of sufficient severity or duration to render a person incapable of working for at least one year. Eligibility is not based on income or resources but on the ability to work. Income becomes important because, as with other unearned sources, it represents an important measure of an individual's ability to work.

Accordingly, people whose average monthly earnings exceed what is termed the *SGA amount* will be deemed able to work, notwithstanding the medical findings. Ordinarily this would result in the cessation of cash benefits and in the loss of Medicare coverage, but the work incentive provisions can ease an often harsh result.

With the TWP, individuals can earn at above the SGA level for nine months, during which time it is determined whether they are actually capable of sustained economic activity. Benefits will not be curtailed until finding at the end of the nine months that the individual is able to work, in which case cash benefits will cease three months later. Medicare can be continued for approximately another two years. This is especially important, perhaps decisive, given the continuing restricted availability of private health insurance to people with disabilities and the decline in the percentage of people covered by employer insurance.

Even when a person deemed able to work earns an average monthly income that exceeds the SGA amount, it need not result in the loss of benefits at the end of the trial work period. This is because in determining income for SGA purposes, sums expended on impairment-work related expenses must be deducted from total earnings. The definition of IRWEs differs slightly from the one we encountered in the Internal Revenue Code for purposes of MS. It is important to note that a wide variety of goods and services essential to and used for work would qualify for IRWE designation, including in many cases medication used for symptom management and suppression in order to facilitate work.

Comparable incentives also exist in many other income replacement and financial assistance programs. In private sector settings such as health or disability insurance, it may also prove possible to negotiate such arrangements with carriers who appreciate the potential financial return on restoration of work but who understand that cooperative relationships among insurers, employers, and beneficiaries are necessary to accomplish this.

MS and other fluctuating conditions inevitably involve practical problems not necessarily associated with more stable disabilities or conditions. They are not insuperable, however. Despite the barriers, the potential for some measure of work with some degree of subsidization seems greater than it has been in the past, particularly for start-up technology or necessary services.

Chapter 7

An Employment Perspective from the National Multiple Sclerosis Society

Gary Sumner

Editor's Note: *Established in 1946, the National Multiple Sclerosis Society is the world's largest advocacy organization for people with MS and their families. The Society's home offices in New York and Denver and its 136 chapters and branches across the United States administer more than $100 million annually to support research, service, educational, and advocacy initiatives. The Society's primary service objective is to promote knowledge about MS, health, and independence for all people whose lives are affected by the disease. A directory of the Society's chapters is presented in Appendix B.*

For people diagnosed with an unpredictable and variable illness such as multiple sclerosis, a matter of paramount concern is how they will financially support themselves and their families. Generally, people with MS are well-educated, have had substantial employment experience, and have been productive in their work. Yet far too many (75–80 percent) of these capable individuals are not utilizing their skills in the employment arena.

Although the question "why do so many people with MS leave the labor force?" has not been definitively answered, many factors have been associated with unemployment among people with MS. As noted in Chapter 2, these include health status, psychological difficulties, work disincentives in the Social Security program, and employer discrimination. With all of these impedi-

National Multiple Sclerosis Society, Client & Community Services Department

ments, it is not surprising that people with MS tend to leave their jobs within a few years of diagnosis.

As if coping with the medical and psychological aspects of MS is not difficult enough, the impact that not working has on a person's self-image makes the illness even more debilitating. When people relinquish the feelings of independence and self-control that go along with productive employment, they become increasingly dependent on caregivers, family members, and benefit systems (e.g., Social Security, long-term disability insurance). This creates a situation wherein capability and potential go unrealized and unfulfilled, and one which thereby deprives the person with MS of the self-sufficiency to which he or she had been accustomed. It also deprives society at large of the contributions that he or she could make as a successful and productive worker.

Employment is, for most people, a very important part of life—certainly more than just an avenue for earning money. What people do vocationally in large part defines their identities and serves as an important component of their value systems. In essence, what we do is who we are in American society, and multiple sclerosis can have a devastating impact on both.

The National Multiple Sclerosis Society has long been committed to providing services to people with MS that enhance their employment opportunities and thereby improve their quality of life. In 1991 the Society formalized its dedication to employment concerns in a detailed position paper, "Employment Issues in Multiple Sclerosis." Twelve principles were given, which provided a foundation and served to guide our employment efforts. Those principles are as follows:

1. Disability in itself should never be assumed to reduce the capability of an individual to work.

2. The Society supports the concepts and principles of the ADA and commits to take a lead role in its implementation.

3. Barrier-free and accessible environments are crucial to maximize employment opportunities for people with disabilities.

4. Small accommodations in the work environment can enable many disabled citizens to be productively employed.

5. Negative attitudes toward the disabled create a major barrier to their employment. Responsibility for changing attitudes must be

shared by business, government, public and private sector agencies, health care providers, the media, labor, educators, and people with disabilities themselves.

6. The Society supports legislative change to remove work disincentives for those with disabilities and advocates implementation policies to help disabled people access their rights under the law.

7. The Society supports legislation that provides incentives to employers to promote the employment of people with disabilities.

8. The Society urges changes in vocational rehabilitation policies that facilitate the employment of people with MS.

9. The Society supports research to benefit those with MS and other disabilities by promoting understanding of work-related issues and identifying solutions to existing problems. This includes the continuing development of technology that will enable people with disabilities to increase their work capabilities. Such technology should be made available and affordable.

10. The Society supports the development of a comprehensive long-term care system that provides social, health, and personal services for all Americans.

11. The Society applauds businesses and organizations that have voluntary plans for significant and special efforts (Affirmative Action) in the recruitment and accommodation of employees with disabilities.

12. Programs and policies that are intended to assist people with disabilities should reflect the thoughts and opinions of those whose lives will be affected by their practices.

Over the past twenty years, the Society has been involved in a number of initiatives to enhance employment opportunities for people with MS and other disabilities. These efforts have included signed agreements with the Rehabilitation Services Administration, the National Institute on Disability and Rehabilitation Research, the Council of State Administrators of Vocational Rehabilitation, and numerous state agencies; Operation Job Match, Job Raising, and Project Alliance (see Chapter 4); and numerous grants from federal and private agencies. Additionally, the Society's Health Services Research program has sponsored a number of employment-related projects to expand the knowledge base concerning the career development implications of MS.

Currently, the Society's primary employment objectives are to assist people with MS in securing and/or maintaining employment, enhancing their employment situations, and obtaining information and support related to the termination of employment if and when that does occur. Additionally, the Society's secondary objectives are to assist employers in increasing their awareness of the legal rights of people with disabilities and of the specific employment concerns of people with MS. All of these objectives are achieved through the following services and activities:

1. *Job development assistance.* Offering programs to provide education to people with MS regarding their legal rights; developing instruments to assess skills, interests, and abilities; and providing placement assistance (resumé preparation, interviewing skills training, structured job search activities, etc.).

2. *Employment retention services.* Interventions with people with MS and their employers to identify barriers to job performance and ways to reduce or remove those barriers, including reasonable accommodations at the worksite.

3. *Educational programs or direct assistance to enhance employment.* Services that focus on such areas as handling disclosure with employers and coworkers, managing symptoms at the workplace, how to implement reasonable accommodations, and maintaining productivity at work.

4. *Information on the termination of employment.* Offering counseling and support related to issues such as Social Security Disability Insurance, work incentives, and maintaining quality of life through meaningful and productive activity.

Since 1946 the National Multiple Sclerosis Society has been dedicated to helping people with MS and their families improve their quality of life. From the body of research described in this book and the wide range of activities described in this chapter, it is clear that employment issues have played a major role in the Society's mission and service delivery.

In spite of many successful initiatives to enhance career prospects for people with MS, the fact remains that too many Americans with multiple sclerosis are unemployed. In collaboration with health care professionals, researchers, rehabilitation practitioners, social workers, people with MS, and their families and friends, we hope to continue our efforts to minimize the impact that MS has on employment, independence, and financial security.

Chapter 8

Policy, Programming, and Research Recommendations

Phillip D. Rumrill, Jr.

This book reflects the considerable compendium of research that has been devoted to the employment implications of multiple sclerosis. As advancements in treatment, symptom management, vocational assessment strategies, placement and retention programs, and federal legislation continue to hold significant promise for members of the MS community and their families and friends, the troubling fact remains that far too few people with MS are presently engaged in the labor force.

Unfortunately, this under-representation is occurring at a time when employers need well-trained, experienced workers more than they have at any point in recent history. According to Mullins, Rumrill, and Roessler (in press), the ever-aging American populace (a function of the "baby boom" generation having fewer children than its parents had and longer life expectancies) will have decreasing numbers of working-age constituents from which to draw over the next three decades. Therefore, they exhorted the rehabilitation profession and the employer community to work together to identify strategies to place, accommodate, and maintain qualified people with disabilities in work roles. Several facts make people with MS an ideal labor pool for employers seeking to meet society's growing need for diversity in the workplace.

1. The vast majority (more than 90 percent) of people with MS have employment histories (LaRocca & Hall, 1990).

2. The onset of the illness typically occurs at around age thirty—usually after the individual has established herself in a career (Kraft, 1981; Rumrill, Battersby, & Kaleta, in press).

3. People with MS are well-educated; most have completed some form of postsecondary training (Roessler & Rumrill, 1995a).

4. Employers report that most workers with MS perform at levels equal to or higher than nondisabled employees (Sumner, 1995).

5. More than half of the accommodations used by employees with MS cost nothing or very little (under $50) to implement (Rumrill, 1993; Roessler & Rumrill, 1995a).

It should be noted that people with MS are not unique among members of the disability community in their ability to succeed in employment. According to the DuPont Corporation (1990, p. 3), among people with disabilities, "[employers] will find a pool of qualified, motivated employees." As early as 1954, for example, long before enactment of the Rehabilitation Act and the Americans with Disabilities Act, a survey of New York City businesses found the performance of employees with disabilities equal to the performance of nondisabled workers (Federation Employment and Guidance Services, 1957). In fact, one-third of employers in that survey rated employees with disabilities as superior workers. In a 1961 study, more than 60 percent of managers and supervisors reported that employees with disabilities were more conscientious about their work and more independent than their nondisabled colleagues (Schletzer, Dawis, England, & Lofquist, 1961).

More recently, findings from DuPont's (1990) thirty-year study of workers with disabilities support the company's prediction that Americans with disabilities will provide a valuable resource for twenty-first century employers. Over the past three decades, 97 percent of DuPont's employees with disabilities were rated average or above in safety. In attendance, 86 percent were rated average or above. In overall job performance, some 90 percent received average or above average ratings. Significantly, these impressive evaluations have not been limited to employees in entry-level or unskilled occupations; nearly half (45 percent) of DuPont's 1990 employees with disabilities held technical, managerial, or professional positions (DuPont Corporation, 1990).

Indeed, people with MS who keep their jobs have proven equal to the task in the workplace. Why, then, do so many leave their jobs, often before the occurrence of severe symptoms? To the extent that researchers have found limited success to date in explaining the high rate of unemployment among people with MS, a more applied, problem-solving focus is warranted. Specifically, the following pages will be used to answer the question, "what can researchers, practitioners, and people with MS themselves do to increase the rate of labor force participation within the American MS community?"

1. Continue the Search for a Cure and Increasingly Effective Treatments.

Although the severity of medical symptoms does not completely determine whether a person with MS will acquire or maintain employment, efforts to minimize or eliminate the effects of the illness can only aid the rehabilitation process. The search for preventive and arrestive cures has been hampered by the elusiveness of the disease's origin (scientists have been unable to determine with certainty how a person develops MS), but recent treatments such as those described in Chapter 1 have shown some promise in alleviating the far-reaching psycho-medical impact of the illness (Rumrill, Battersby, & Kaleta, in press).

Illness and disability prevention initiatives have not always met with unanimous favor among disability groups. In *No Pity*, an excellent historical account of the "disability rights" movement in the United States, Shapiro (1993) noted that many disability advocates oppose medical research that seeks to cure existing disabling conditions. The argument against such measures is that they degrade and dehumanize people who already have those conditions, and that they could deprive people of the opportunity to have a disability. Certain groups have gone so far as to challenge mandatory seat belt and lower speed limit laws (which decrease spinal cord and traumatic brain injuries), early prenatal screenings for potential birth defects, and cochlear implants for people who are deaf, suggesting that these measures stand to reduce the constituency and consequent strength of the disability community.

This author does not share these views. Multiple sclerosis research directed at finding a cure and refining treatments must continue. Efforts to prevent or treat disabilities do not preclude acceptance of people who have those disabilities, and I believe that most people with MS—even those who have effectively adjusted to the illness—would prefer not to have developed the disease in the first place. Hence, people's prospects for increased independence, the abiding mission of both the disability rights movement and the vocational rehabilitation process, will be enhanced, not hindered, by future medical advancements in MS research.

2. Target Members of Traditionally Underserved Populations Who Have MS

To the extent that minority status presents an inherent disadvantage in the career development process in the general population (Zunker, 1994), it seems logical that coupling MS with membership in a traditionally underserved group could pose a "double obstacle" to employment success. It has been documented that women, who comprise a decided majority of the American MS community, find it more difficult to maintain employment while coping with the illness than do men (Kornblith, LaRocca, & Baum, 1986; LaRocca et al., 1985). Also experiencing particular difficulty are people with MS whose occupations require less education and demand significant physical exertion (Ketelaer et al., 1993). Accordingly, special effort should be made to direct employment initiatives such as those described in Chapter 4 toward those people with MS who need them the most. In addition to women and people with lower educational attainment, these "high need" groups may include people of color (although the worldwide MS population is predominantly white), individuals who reside in rural areas, and people who do not have successful employment histories.

3. Focus on Success: What Factors Enable People with MS to Keep Their Jobs?

The majority of research on the employment of people with disabilities focuses on the difficulties that people encounter in every stage of the career development process. Even in this book, much of the focus has been placed on such negative aspects of the world of work as unemployment, on-the-job barriers, functional decrements, and psychological problems. What about the people with MS who successfully maintain employment? What can researchers, practitioners, and people with MS learn from them to help those who are confronted with the difficulties noted here? People with MS comprise a qualified, capable, and seasoned labor resource, and people seeking to actualize their talents can learn a great deal from their community leaders, support group members, and friends who have MS, and who have successfully negotiated the rigors and uncertainty of working with an unpredictable, chronic illness.

4. Encourage Utilization of Vocational Rehabilitation Services

The fact that people with MS underutilize vocational rehabilitation services does not mean that they are disproportionally ineligible for those services. Even people with MS whose disabilities are not "severe" enough to render them eligible for paid services can receive valuable personal consultation and referral services from vocational rehabilitation agencies. Physicians, nurses, social workers, and other service providers must refer their patients and clients with MS (especially those dealing with the most severe symptoms) to the vocational rehabilitation program as a matter of course.

5. Develop Early Intervention Strategies to Help People with MS Keep Their Jobs

To the extent that the most precipitous decline in physical functioning typically occurs during the first five years after diagnosis of MS (Gulick & Bugg, 1992), recently diagnosed people (the majority of whom are employed) may need assistance with such on-the-job issues as when and how to disclose any disability-related work limitations, identifying how those limitations could be overcome via reasonable accommodations, and requesting accommodations from their employers as per Title I of the ADA (Roessler & Rumrill, 1994b, 1995a; Rumrill, 1993). Unfortunately, these pressing needs for employment assistance occur at a time when a considerable portion of the person's energy is being devoted to psychological adjustment to the disease itself (Marsh, Ellison, & Strite, 1983), reassessment of other social roles, learning more about the disease, and symptom management. With all of these considerations, it is understandable that employment may not be the person's most prominent concern during the early stages of MS. However, to the extent that career identity constitutes a defining attribute for many people (what one does for work is who one is), the issue of work must be addressed as part of the person's medical, personal, and social orientation to MS.

Specifically, health care professionals, social workers, psychologists, and rehabilitation professionals must work closely with local chapters of the National Multiple Sclerosis Society and other consumer advocacy groups to provide coordinated, early-intervention support for people with MS. Many chapters offer "newly diagnosed" support groups, and the vocational implications of MS should be systematically addressed in those programs. Finally, physicians are exhorted to refrain from prescribing unemployment as a treatment strategy. The therapeutic benefits of working (not to mention the potentially devastating psychological impact of not working) make it imperative for responsible practitioners to encourage anyone who wants to work to continue to do so. If and when the person with MS chooses to stop working, that decision must be hers and hers alone.

6. *Provide Ongoing Employment Assistance: Early Interventions Are Necessary But Not Sufficient*

The difficulties associated with maintaining employment while coping with a disability are by no means unique to people with multiple sclerosis. In fact, studies show that people with disabilities in general need more support in the job retention process than is presently available within existing service delivery mechanisms.

Roessler and Bolton (1985) documented a "lateral movement phenomenon" in their follow-up survey of fifty-seven former vocational rehabilitation clients with various disabilities. Career patterns of respondents consisted primarily of changes from one entry-level job to another, often interspersed with extended periods of unemployment. Neubert, Tilson, and Ianacone (1989) also substantiated the problems that people with disabilities have in holding jobs following initial placement. Their study of sixty-six people with disabilities who had completed a postsecondary transition program revealed an encouraging 68 percent employment rate at a one-year follow-up. However, 36 percent of those participants who were employed had not been continuously employed for the entire one-year period. Moreover, participants' occupational changes during the follow-up period tended to follow Roessler and Bolton's (1985) lateral pattern.

Perhaps the most compelling rationale for increased post-employment services for people with disabilities can be drawn from data reported by Gibbs (1990). In a follow-up survey of

2,536 former vocational rehabilitation clients whose cases had been closed by virtue of successful employment, Gibbs found initial periods of employment of less than three months among some 25 percent of respondents. One year after case closure, only 51 percent were still employed. During Gibbs's 54-month tracking period, no less than 84.4 percent of these successful rehabilitants experienced some interruption of employment, and many were never re-employed.

Indeed, although the vocational rehabilitation program (the nation's oldest and largest service system for people with disabilities) purports to "rehabilitate" more than half of its clients, it appears to have a short-term (at best) impact on clients' abilities to work and live independently. Two years after "successful" case closure, rehabilitants' mean income drops below the income that they reported at the time of enrollment in the vocational rehabilitation program. (United States General Accounting Office (1993).

From these findings, it should be clear that people with multiple sclerosis are not alone in their need for effective and comprehensive post-employment services. However, the unpredictable, often episodic nature of the illness does warrant special consideration on the part of employees, employers, and service providers alike. On-the-job interventions that address the employee's unique and often fluctuating needs must be available on an ongoing, as-needed basis if the person with MS is to maintain and fully succeed in his career.

7. Encourage Self-Advocacy and Consumer Involvement

With the fairly recent enactment of the ADA and a growing societal commitment to include people with disabilities in every aspect of life, people with MS and other disabilities are being expected to take a more active role in society than ever before. As mainstream structures and institutions continue to reduce the barriers to inclusion, active involvement stands to become less of a concession to people with disabilities and more of a requirement for them. The provisions of the ADA, for example, call for a great deal of initiative on the part of individuals with disabilities in asserting their civil rights to accessible employment opportunities, public services, public accommodations, and communication systems.

With respect to employment, Title I of the ADA (see Chapter 5) requires the person with a disability to take an active role in

(1) requesting reasonable accommodations from her employer, (2) identifying resources that can facilitate the accommodation process, and (3) monitoring the ongoing effectiveness of on-the-job accommodations (Equal Employment Opportunity Commission & Department of Justice, 1991). It also requires those who have experienced employment discrimination to file a formal complaint and follow a series of administrative and legal procedures. Hence, people with MS need accurate information about their rights under the ADA. They may also require individual or group consultation concerning the often complicated nuances of civil rights law and how to access the protections to which they are entitled.

8. Make Employment a Priority: No One Is "Too Disabled" to Work

Some experts have suggested that the woeful rate of labor force participation among Americans with disabilities is attributable in part to the fact that society "excuses" people whom it considers unable to work (Schriner, Rumrill, & Parlin, 1994, 1995). However, the idea of a person being "too disabled" to work has come under fire recently. Research indicates that the severity of a person's disability has little bearing on his prospects for successful rehabilitation; rather, such factors as motivation and residual abilities are more predictive of success (Rubin & Roessler, 1995). Accordingly, many contemporary job placement and retention programs are predicated on the assumption that anyone who wants to work can work and should be encouraged to do so to every extent possible—regardless of disability (Rumrill & Gordon, 1994).

To make employment a viable option for people diagnosed with MS, service providers, family members, and friends must reinforce the expectation that people can stay on their jobs as long as they want to. By expecting success and orienting themselves toward functional abilities and capacities (rather than focusing on DYSfunction, DISability, and INcapacitation), people with MS will be much more likely to retain and advance in their jobs.

9. Consult Assistive Technology Resources

Another promising factor in helping people with MS to retain and advance in their jobs is the use of appropriate assistive technology. As developmental advancements continue in this area, people with MS and other disabilities stand to be more independent, more productive in daily living and employment capacities, and less susceptible to the functional limitations associated with their conditions. Most states have federally sponsored technology assistance programs designed to help people with disabilities in identifying, acquiring, and learning to use assistive devices. Appendix D presents a state-by-state directory of those programs.

10. Conduct Research with Broad-Based National Samples

Employment interventions and other initiatives designed to increase the knowledge base concerning the career development implications of MS must be implemented at the national level. Far too many of the studies described in Chapters 2, 3, and 4 involved "micro-samples" that were restricted to circumscribed geographic areas. Multisite projects such as the Career Possibilities Project, the Job Raising Program, and Project Alliance need to be adopted on an ongoing, systematic basis.

In particular, a scientifically derived national sample of Americans with MS needs to be surveyed as to the employment-related concerns people with MS have in the ADA era. The field needs up-to-date information about (1) labor force participation, (2) predictors of employment status, (3) the effect of Betaseron® and other newly developed treatments on employment, and (4) the extent to which members of the MS community are utilizing the civil rights protections of the ADA. Perhaps most importantly, a thorough investigation of respondents' self-reported employment concerns would enable researchers and service providers to develop interventions that are truly compatible with the needs of the MS community.

Multiple sclerosis is an unpredictable disease that presents a wide range of adjustmental challenges for those who develop the illness. Typically occurring during the prime of life, MS disrupts and often impairs the person's ability to plan for the future, perform activities of daily living, work, and engage in virtually every other social role. Although the medical effects of MS are many, varied, and often severe, the capricious disease course and associated psychological impact make the illness a doubly difficult one to cope with, adjust to, and accept.

These factors combine to create a unique and imposing challenge for people with MS who wish to continue working. As a group, people with MS are well-educated, experienced, and productive employees, yet a high percentage make a premature departure from the labor force.

To the extent that existing service delivery mechanisms (e.g., vocational rehabilitation, independent living centers, workers' compensation) have had little success to date in addressing the complex career development needs of people with MS, researchers and service providers must join together to:

1. Further specify the seemingly unique impact that MS has on a person's employment prospects;

2. Develop interventions to address those needs in a way that enables the person herself to take primary responsibility for her ultimate employment success; and

3. Evaluate the effectiveness of those programs on a systematic, ongoing basis.

The purpose of this book is to detail the medical, demographic, psychological, and social factors that affect the employment status of people with MS. It also seeks to describe model assessment and intervention strategies that have demonstrated the potential to assist people with MS in seeking, securing, and maintaining employment. Coupling that information with knowledge of the Americans with Disabilities Act, tax benefits and work incentives, and the resources of service organizations such as the National Multiple Sclerosis Society will afford people with MS the best opportunity to establish and continue in their careers, thereby enabling them to enjoy the well-documented economic, personal, and social benefits of active participation in the world of work.

Appendix A

Selected Resources and References: Social Security, Workers' Compensation, and Long-Term Disability

(Roessler & Farley, 1993, pp. 78–79)

1. Social Security
   a. Contact the Regional Social Security Claims Office in your area.
   b. "Red Book on Work Incentives—A Summary Guide to Social Security and Supplemental Security Income Work Incentives for the Disabled and Blind," Social Security Administration, Office of Disability, SSA, Pub. #64-030, IC/U 436900, June 1991.
   c. Szymanski E (1988). Rehabilitation planning with Social Security Work Incentives: A sequential guide for the rehabilitation professional. *Journal of Rehabilitation* 54(2):28–33.

2. Workers' Compensation
   a. Analysis of Workers' Compensation Laws, prepared and published annually by the U.S. Chamber of Commerce, 1616 H Street, NW, Washington, D.C. 20062 (301-468-5128).
   b. Contact the Regional Office of U.S. Department of Labor for federal jurisdictions of Workers' Compensation.
   c. Commercial Insurance Carriers Claims Department, Claims Supervisor or Claims Manager.
   d. Contact the Industrial Commission in your state for a copy of the State Compensation Act and for consultation.
   e. State Bar Association or Trial Lawyers Association.

    f. Local chapter of the National Association of Rehabilitation Practitioners in the Private Sector (NARPPS).

    g. State or local Chamber of Commerce.

3. Long-Term Disability Insurance

    a. Consult individual and group policies.

    b. Consult claims personnel or legal advisor if applicable.

    c. Consult employee benefits manager if employer sponsored a group plan.

Appendix B

Chapters of the National Multiple Sclerosis Society

Alabama Chapter
3125 Montgomery Highway,
  #303
Birmingham, AL 35209
(205) 879–8881

Alaska Chapter
511 West 41st Avenue, Ste. 101
Anchorage, AK 99503–6643
(907) 562–6673

Desert Southwest Chapter
P.O. Box 61654
Phoenix, AZ 85082
(602) 277–8459

Arkansas Chapter
1100 N. University Place,
  Ste. 225
Evergreen Place
Little Rock, AR 72207
(501) 663–6767

Central California Chapter
770 East Shaw, #222
Fresno, CA 93710
(209) 226–2005

Southern California Chapter
230 N. Maryland Avenue,
  Ste. 303
Glendale, CA 91206–4261
(818) 247–1175

Northern California Chapter
150 Grand Avenue
Oakland, CA 94612
(510) 268–0572

Orange County Chapter
17752 Mitchell, Ste. F
Irvine, CA 92714
(714) 752–1680

Mountain Valley Calif. Chapter
2277 Watt Avenue, Ste. A
Sacramento, CA 95825
(916) 486–8981

San Diego Area Chapter
4715 Viewridge Avenue, Ste. 150
San Diego, CA 92123
(619) 974–8640

Channel Islands Chapter
3022–A De La Vina
Santa Barbara, CA 93105
(805) 682–8783

Santa Clara County Chapter
2589 Scott Boulevard
Santa Clara, CA 95050
(408) 988–7557

Colorado Chapter
1777 S. Harrison Street, Ste. 200
Denver, CO 80210
(303) 691–2956

Greater Connecticut Chapter
1155 Silas Deane Highway
Wethersfield, CT 06109
(203) 721–6001

Western Connecticut Chapter
83 East Avenue, Ste. 113
Norwalk, CT 06851
(203) 838–1033

Delaware Chapter
Two Mill Road, Ste. 106
Wilmington, DE 19806
(302) 655–5610

National Capitol Chapter
2021 K Street NW, Ste. 100
Washington, D.C. 20006
(202) 296–5363

Central Florida Chapter
3191 Maguire Boulevard,
   Ste. 185
Orlando, FL 32803
(407) 896–3873

Florida Gulf Coast Chapter
200 South Hoover Boulevard
Bldg. 215, Ste. 120
Tampa, FL 33609
(813) 287–2939

North Florida Chapter
9550 Regency Square Boulevard,
   Ste. 104
Jacksonville, FL 32225
(904) 725–6800

South Florida Chapter
5410 NW 33rd Avenue, Ste. 108
Fort Lauderdale, FL 33309
(305) 731–4224

Georgia Chapter
1100 Circle 75 Parkway,
   Ste. 630
Atlanta, GA 30339
(770) 984–9080

Hawaii Chapter
245 North Kukui Street, #104
Honolulu, HI 96817
(808) 531–4127

Idaho Chapter
6901 Emerald, Ste. 203
Boise, ID 83704
(208) 322–6721

Chicago–Greater Illinois Chapter
600 South Federal Street,
   Ste. 204
Chicago, IL 60605
(312) 922–8000

Indiana State Chapter
615 N. Alabama Street,
   Rm. 318
Indianapolis, IN 46204
(317) 634–8796

Iowa Chapter
2400 86th Street, Ste. 29
Des Moines, IA 50322
(515) 270–6337

So. Central & W. Kansas Chapter
250 South Laura
Wichita, KS 67211
(316) 264–1333

Kentucky Chapter
835 West Jefferson Street,
   Ste. 105
Louisville, KY 40202
(502) 587–6767

Louisiana Chapter
3616 South I–10 Service Road,
   Ste. 101
Metairie, LA 70001
(504) 832–4013

Maine Chapter
P.O. Box 8730
Portland, ME 04104
(207) 761–5815

Maryland Chapter
1055 Taylor Avenue,
    Ste. 201
Towson, MD 21286–8327
(410) 821–8626

Massachusetts Chapter
101 First Avenue, Ste. 6
Waltham, MA 02154–1115
(617) 890–4990

Michigan Chapter
26111 Evergreen, Ste. 100
Southfield, MI 48076
(810) 350–0020

Minnesota North Star Chapter
2344 Nicollet Avenue
Minneapolis, MN 55404
(612) 870–1500

Mississippi Chapter
P.O. Box 390
Jackson, MS 39205
(601) 981–5364

Mid–America Chapter
P.O. Box 2292
Shawnee Mission, KS 66201
(913) 432–3926

Gateway Area Chapter
14 Sunnen Drive, Ste. 143
Maplewood, MO 63143
(314) 781–9020

Montana Chapter
1601 2nd Avenue North
Great Falls, MT 59401
(406) 452–9529

Midlands Chapter
Community Health Plaza
7101 Newport Avenue,
    Ste. 203
Omaha, NE 68152–2160
(402) 572–3190

Great Basin Sierra Chapter
3100 Mill Street, #115
Reno, NV 89502
(702) 329–7180

New Hampshire Chapter
27 Harvey Road
Bedford, NH 03110
(603) 623–3501

Greater North Jersey Chapter
P.O. Box 1606
Paramus, NJ 07653
(201) 967–5599

Mid–Jersey Chapter
801 Belmar Plaza
Belmar, NJ 07719
(908) 681–2322

Rio Grande Chapter
2021 Girard S.E., Ste. 112
Albuquerque, NM 87106
(505) 842–6767

Northeastern New York Chapter
324 Broadway, 4th Floor
Albany, NY 12207–2977
(518) 427–0421

South Central New York Chapter
32 West State Street, 1st Floor
Binghamton, NY 13901
(607) 724–5464

Long Island Chapter
200 Parkway Drive South, #101
Hauppauge, NY 11788
(516) 864–8837

New York City Chapter
30 West 26th Street, 9th Floor
New York, NY 10010–2094
(212) 463–7787

Rochester Area Chapter
1000 Elmwood Avenue
Rochester, NY 14620
(716) 271–0801

Upstate New York Chapter
404 Oak Street
Syracuse, NY 13203
(315) 422–1447

Southern New York Chapter
11 Skyline Drive
Hawthorne, NY 10532
(914) 345–3500

W. New York/N.W. Penn. Chapter
2060 Sheridan Drive
Buffalo, NY 14223
(716) 875–7710

Central North Carolina Chapter
2302 W. Meadowview Road,
   Ste. 101
Greensboro, NC 27407–3700
(910) 299–4136

Greater Carolinas Chapter
1515 Mockingbird Lane,
   Ste. 1000
Charlotte, NC 28209
(704) 525–2955

Eastern N. Carolina Chapter
3725 National Drive, Ste. 125
Raleigh, NC 27612–4879
(919) 781–0676

Dakota Chapter
2801 Main Avenue
Fargo, ND 58103
(701) 235–2678

Northeast Ohio Chapter
The Hanna Building
1422 Euclid Avenue, Ste. 333
Cleveland, OH 44115–1901
(216) 696–8220

Mid–Ohio Chapter
1550 Old Henderson Rd.,
   W–101
Columbus, OH 43220
(614) 459–2220

S.W. Ohio/N. Kentucky Chapter
4460 Lake Forest Drive,
   Ste. 236
Cincinnati, OH 45242
(513) 769–4400

Western Ohio Chapter
The Woolpert Building
409 E. Monument, Ste. 101
Dayton, OH 45402
(513) 461–5232

Northwest Ohio Chapter
415 Tomahawk Drive
Maumee, OH 43537
(419) 897–9533

Oklahoma Chapter
4606 East 67th Street,
   Ste. 201
Building #7
Tulsa, OK 74136
(918) 488–0882

Oregon Chapter
5901 S.W. Macadam, Ste. 100
Portland, OR 97201
(503) 223–9511

Central Pennsylvaniá Chapter
2209 Forest Hills Drive, #18
Harrisburg, PA 17112–1005
(717) 652–2108

Greater Delaware Valley Chapter
1 Reed Street
Philadelphia, PA 19147
(215) 271–1500

Allegheny District Chapter
1040 Fifth Avenue, 2nd Floor
Pittsburgh, PA 15219
(412) 261–6347

Rhode Island Chapter
535 Centerville Road
Warwick, RI 02886
(401) 738–8383

Setenga Chapter
6100 Bldg.—Eastgate Center,
  Ste. 4800
Chattanooga, TN 37411
(615) 954–9700

Middle Tennessee Chapter
4219 Hillsboro Road, Ste. 306
Nashville, TN 37215
(615) 269–9055

Mid–South Chapter
755 Crossover Lane
Building A, Ste. 101
Memphis, TN 38117
(901) 763–3601

South Texas Chapter
140 Heimer #195
San Antonio, TX 78232
(210) 494–5531

North Texas Chapter
8750 North Central Expressway,
  Ste. 1030
Dallas, TX 75231
(214) 373–1400

North Central Texas Chapter
5017 South Hulen Street,
  Ste. 6
Fort Worth, TX 76132–1936
(817) 263–8200

Southeast Texas Chapter
2211 Norfolk, Ste. 825
Houston, TX 77098
(713) 526–8967

Panhandle Chapter
715 South Lamar
Amarillo, TX 79106
(806) 372–4429

West Texas Chapter
P.O. Box 4636
Midland, TX 79704
(915) 684–4097

Utah State Chapter
525 South 300 West
Salt Lake City, UT 84101
(801) 575–8500

Vermont Chapter
Champlain Mill #42
1 Main Street
Winooski, VT 05404
(802) 655–3666

Blue Ridge Chapter
P.O. Box 6808
Charlottesville, VA 22906
(804) 971–8010

Central Virginia Chapter
1301 North Hamilton Street,
  Ste. 108
Richmond, VA 23230–3959
(804) 353–5008

Hampton Roads Chapter
405 S. Parliament Drive,
  Ste. 105
Virginia Beach, VA 23462
(804) 490–9627

Inland Northwest Chapter
818 East Sharp
Spokane, WA 99202
(509) 482–2022

Western Washington Chapter
192 Nickerson Street,
  Ste. 100
Seattle, WA 98109
(206) 284–4236

Central Washington Chapter
P.O. Box 1093
Yakima, WA 98907
(509) 248–2350

West Virginia Chapter
4825 Maccorkle Avenue S.W.
South Charleston, WV 25309
(304) 768–9775

Wisconsin Chapter
W224 N608 Saratoga Dr., Ste. 110
Waukesha, WI 53186–0401
(414) 547–8999

Wyoming Chapter
P.O. Box 556
Casper, WY 82602
(307) 234–2340

Puerto Rico Chapter
P.O. Box 29085
San Jaun, PR 00929–0085
(809) 763–0303

Appendix C

Selected Disability Resources

General

Clearinghouse on Disability Information
Office of Special Education &
   Rehab Services
U.S. Department of Education

Switzer Building, Rm. 3232
Washington, D.C. 20202-2524
202–732–1723 (voice/TTD)

Health Resource Center

One DuPont Circle #800
Washington, D.C. 20036–1193
800–544–3284

National Easter Seal Society

70 East Lake Street
Chicago, IL 60601
312–726–6200

National Organization on Disability

910 16th Street, NW, Rm. 600
Washington, D.C. 20006
1–800–248–ABLE

World Institute on Disability

510 16th Street
Oakland, CA 94612
415–736–4100

ADA Legal

ADA Clearinghouse and Resource
   Center
National Center for State Courts

300 Newport Avenue
Williamsburg, VA 23185
804–253–2000

American Bar Association
Commission on Mental & Physical
   Disability Law

1800 M Street, NW
Washington, D.C. 20036
202–331–2240

Disability Rights Education &
   Defense Fund

2121 Sixth Street
Berkeley, CA 94710
800–466–4ADA

Social Security Administration

6401 Security Boulevard
Baltimore, MD 21202
800–772–1213

Employment

The Association for Persons in
Supported Employment

5001 W. Broad Street, Ste. 34
Richmond, VA 23230
804–282–3655

Foundation on Employment and
Disability

3820 Del Amo Blvd, #201
Torrance, CA 90503
213–214–3430

Goodwill Industries of America, Inc.

9200 W. Wisconsin Avenue
Bethesda, MD 20814–3896
301–530–6500

Job Training Partnership Act (JTPA)
Programs
Office of Job Training Programs
U.S. Department of Labor

200 Constitution Avenue, NW
Rm. N4709
Washington, D.C. 20210
202–535–0580

National Clearinghouse of Rehabilitation
Training Materials

Oklahoma State University
816 West 6th Street
Stillwater, OK 74078
405–624–6200

The President's Committee on
Employment of People with
Disabilities

1331 F Street, NW
Washington, D.C. 20004
202–376–6200

State Vocational Rehabilitation Services
Program
Rehabilitation Services Administration
Office of Special Education & Rehab
Services
U.S. Department of Education

Switzer Building
300 C Street, SW, Rm. 3127
Washington, D.C. 20202–2531
202–732–1282 (voice/TTD)

U.S. Employment Service
Employment and Training Administration
Department of Labor

200 Consultation Avenue, NW
Washington, D.C. 20210
202–535–0189

Vocational Evaluation & Work
Adjustment Assoc.
Div. of the National Rehabilitation.
Assoc.

1910 Association Drive, Ste. 205
Reston, VA 22091
703–636–9306

Technology

Accent on Information	P.O. Box 700 Bloomington, IL 309–378–2961
Center for Computer Assistance to the Disabled (C–CAD)	617 Seventh Avenue Fort Worth, TX 76104 817–870–9082
Center for Rehabilitation Technology (CRT)	Georgia Institute of Tech College of Architecture Atlanta, GA 30332–0156
Direct Link for the Disabled	P.O. Box 1036 Solvang, CA 93464 805–688–1603
IBM National Support Center for Persons with Disabilities	P.O. Box 2150 Atlanta, GA 30055

Sources:

Equal Employment Opportunity Commission (1992). *Technical assistance manual on the employment provisions (Title I) of the Americans with Disabilities Act.* Washington, D.C: Government Printing Office.

Roessler RT, Rumrill P. (1994). *Enhancing productivity on your job: The "win–win" approach to reasonable accommodations.* New York: National Multiple Sclerosis Society.

Appendix D

State Technology Assistance Projects

Statewide Technology Access and Response (STAR) System for Alabamians with Disabilities
Alabama Department of Rehabilitation Services
2129 East South Boulevard
P.O. Box 11586
Montgomery, AL 36111-0586
(205) 288-0240

Alaska Assistive Technology Project
Department of Education
Division of Vocational Rehabilitation
Assistive Technologies of Alaska
400 D Street, Ste. 230
Anchorage, AK 99501
(800) 770-0138

Arizona Technology Access Program (AzTAP)
Northern Arizona University
Arizona University Affiliated Program
2600 North Wyatt Drive
Tucson, AZ 85712
(602) 324-3170

Arkansas ICAN (Increasing Capabilities Access Network)
Department of Education
Vocational Education Division
Arkansas Rehabilitation Services
2201 Brookwood Drive, Ste. 117
Little Rock, AR 72202
(800) 828-2799

California Assistive Technology System (CATS)
Department of Rehabilitation
Independent Living Division
830 K Street
Sacramento, CA 95814
(916) 327-3967

Colorado Assistive Technology Project: Developing Colorado's
   Consumer Responsive System
Rocky Mountain Resource and Training Institute
6355 Ward Road, Ste. 310
Arvada, CO 80004
(303) 420-2942

Connecticut Assistive Technology Program
Connecticut Department of Social Services
Bureau of Rehabilitation Services
10 Griffin Road North
Windsor, CT 06095
(203) 298-9590

Delaware Assistive Technology Initiative (DATI)
University of Delaware
Center for Applied Science and Engineering
A.I. duPont Institute
1600 Rockland Road
P.O. Box 269
Wilmington, DE 19899
(302) 651-6793

District of Columbia Partnership for Assistive Technology (DCPAT)
District of Columbia Department of Human Services
National Rehabilitation Hospital—Rehabilitation Engineering Dept.
801 Pennsylvania Avenue SE, Ste. 210
Washington, D.C. 20003
(202) 546-9163

Florida's Alliance for Assistive Services and Technology (FAAST)
Florida Department of Labor and Employment Security
Division of Vocational Rehabilitation
2002 Old St. Augustine Road, Building A
Tallahassee, FL 32399-0696
(904) 488-8380

Tools for Life—Georgia Assistive Technology Program
Georgia Department of Human Resources
Division of Rehabilitation Services
2 Peachtree Street NW, Ste. 23-411
Atlanta, GA 30303-3166
(800) 497-8665

Hawaii Assistive Technology System for Persons with Disabilities
Vocational Rehabilitation and Services for the Blind Division
1000 Bishop Street, Rm. 605
Honolulu, HI 96813
(808) 586-5375

Idaho Assistive Technology Project
Idaho Center on Developmental Disabilities
University of Idaho
Professional Building, 129 West Third Street
Moscow, ID 83844-4401
(208) 885-3559

Technology-Related Assistance for Individuals with Disabilities
Illinois Assistive Technology Project
110 Iles Park Place
Springfield, IL 62718
(217) 522-9966

Technology-Related Assistance for Individuals with Disabilities
ATTAIN
402 West Washington Street
P.O. Box 7083
Indianapolis, IN 46207-7083
(800) 545-7763

Iowa Program for Assistive Technology
Rm. 217 UHS
University of Iowa
Iowa City, IA 52242
(800) 331-3027

Assistive Technology for Kansas
University of Kansas
University Affiliated Program at Parsons
Assistive Technology Center
2601 Gabriel

P.O. Box 738
Parsons, KS 67357
(316) 421-8367

The Kentucky Assistive Technology (KATS) Network
Kentucky Department for the Blind
KATS Network Coordinating Center
427 Versailles Road
Frankfort, KY 40601
(502) 573-4665

Louisiana Assistive Technology Access Network (LATAN)
Louisiana State Planning Council for Developmental Disabilities
P.O. Box 3455, Bin 14
1201 Capitol Access Road
Baton Rouge, LA 70821-3455
(800) 922-3425

Maine Consumer Information and Technology Training
    Exchange (Maine CITE)
Maine Department of Education
Division of Special Services
State House Station #23
Augusta, ME 04333

Maryland Technology Assistance Program (MTAP)
Governor's Office for Individuals with Disabilities
MD TAP
Box 10, One Market Center
300 West Lexington Street
Baltimore, MD 21201
(800) 832-4827

Massachusetts Commission for the Deaf and Hard of Hearing
600 Washington Street, Rm. 600
Boston, MA 02111
(617) 735-7820

TECH 2000: Michigan's Assistive Technology Project
Michigan Rehabilitation Services
Community Development Division
P.O. Box 30010
Lansing, MI 48909
(517) 373-4058

A System of Technology to Achieve Results (STAR)
State of Minnesota
Governor's Advisory Council on Technology for People with
  Disabilities
300 Centennial Building
658 Cedar Street
St. Paul, MN 55155
(612) 296-9478

Project START—Success Through Assistive/Rehabilitative
  Technology
Department of Human Services
Office of Vocational Rehabilitation
P.O. Box 1000
Jackson, MS 39215
(800) 852-8328

Missouri Assistive Technology Project
Missouri Department of Labor & Industrial Relations
Governor's Committee on Employment of People with
  Disabilities
4731 South Cochise, Ste. 114
Independence, MO 64055-6975
(800) 647-8557

MonTECH
Montana Department of Social and Rehabilitation Services
Rehabilitative Services Division
111 Sanders
P.O. Box 4210
Helena, MT 59604
(800) 732-0323

Technology-Related Assistance Project
Nebraska Department of Education
Division of Vocational Rehabilitation
301 Centennial Mall South
P.O. Box 94987
Lincoln, NE 68509-4987
(402) 471-0117

Assistive Technology Services, Advocacy, and Systems Change
Nevada Rehabilitation Division

Community-Based Services
711 South Stewart Street
Carson City, NV 89710
(702) 687-4452

Supporting People with Disabilities Through New Hampshire's
Technology Partnership
Institute on Disability
10 Ferry Street, Ste. 307, Unit 14
Concord, NH 03301
(603) 224-0630

Technology Assistive Resource Program
New Jersey Department of Labor
Division of Vocational Rehabilitation Services
CN 398, 135 East State Street, 1st Floor
Trenton, NJ 08625
(800) 382-7765

New Mexico Technology-Related Assistance Program (NMTAP)
State Department of Education
Division of Vocational Rehabilitation
435 Saint Michaels Drive, Building D
Sante Fe, NM 87505
(800) 866-2253

Technology-Related Assistance of Individuals with Disabilities
(TRAID)
New York State Office of Advocate for Persons with Disabilities
TRAID Project
One Empire State Plaza, Ste. 1001
Albany, NY 12223-1150
(800) 522-4369

North Carolina Assistive Technology Project
North Carolina Department of Human Resources
Division of Vocational Rehabilitation Services
1110 Navaho Drive, Ste. 101
Raleigh, NC 27609
(800) 852-0042

Comprehensive Statewide Program of Technology-Related
Assistance for Individuals with Disabilities
North Dakota Department of Human Services

Office of Vocational Rehabilitation
P.O. Box 743
Cavalier, ND 58220
(701) 265-4807

Ohio Project on Technology-Related Assistance for Individuals
  with Disabilities (Ohio T.R.A.I.D.—Tech Act Project)
Ohio State University Research Foundation
Ohio T.R.A.I.N.
Ohio Super Computer Center
1224 Kinnear Road
Columbus, OH 43212
(614) 292-2426

Oklahoma Assistive Technology Program
Oklahoma Department of Rehabilitation
P.O. Box 36659
Oklahoma City, OK 73136
(405) 424-4311, ext. 2722

Technology Access for Life Needs
Department of Human Resources
Vocational Rehabilitation Division
TALN
Chemeketa Community College
4000 Lancaster Drive NE
P.O. Box 14007
Salem, OR 97309-7070
(800) 677-7512

Pennsylvania's Initiative on Assistive Technology
Temple University
Institute on Disabilities/UAP
Ritter Annex, Rm. 433
Philadelphia, PA 19122
(800) 204-PIAT

Rhode Island Assistive Technology Access Partnership (ATAP)
Rhode Island Department of Human Services
Office of Rehabilitation Services
40 Fountain Street
Providence, RI 02903-1898
(401) 421-7005

South Carolina Assistive Technology Program
South Carolina Vocational Rehabilitation Department
P.O. Box 15
1410-C Boston Avenue
West Columbia, SC 29171-0015
(800) 922-1107

DakotaLink
State of South Dakota
Department of Human Services/Division of Rehabilitation
East Highway 34, Hillsview Plaza
c/o 500 East Capitol
Pierre, SD 57501-5070
(800) 645-0673

Tennessee Technology Access Project
Department of Mental Health and Mental Retardation
Tennessee Technology Access
Gateway Plaza, 11th Floor
710 James Robertson Parkway
Nashville, TN 37243-0381
(800) 732-5059

Texas Assistive Technology Partnership Project
Texas Consortium for Developmental Disabilities/AUAP
The University of Texas at Austin
Department of Special Education, EDB, Rm. 306
Austin, TX 78712-1290
(800) 828-7839

Utah Assistive Technology Program (UATP)
Utah State University
Utah Center for Assistive Technology (UCAT)
Center for Persons with Disabilities
UMC 6800
Logan, UT 84322-6855
(801) 797-2153

Technical Assistance Contract
RESNA
1700 North Moore Street, Ste. 1540
Arlington, VA 22209-1903
(703) 524-6686

Assistive Technology Development Grant
Vermont Assistive Technology Project
Department of Aging and Disabilities
103 South Main Street
Waterbury, VT 05676
(800) 639-1522

Virginia Assistive Technology
Department of Rehabilitative Services
VAT
8004 Franklin Farms Drive
Richmond, VA 23288-0300
(800) 435-8490

Washington Assistive Technology Project
Division of Vocational Rehabilitation
Department of Social and Health Services
University of Washington Affiliated Programs
Washington Department of Services for the Blind
P.O. Box 45340
Olympia, WA 98504-5340
(206) 438-8051

Technology-Related Assistance for Individuals with Disabilities:
    WisTech
Wisconsin Department of Health and Social Services
Division of Vocational Rehabilitation
P.O. Box 7852
Madison, WI 53717-7852
(608) 266-1281

West Virginia Assistive Technology System (WVATS)
West Virginia Division of Rehabilitation Services
Capitol Complex
Charleston, WV 25305-0890
(800) 841-8436

Wyoming's New Options in Technology (WYNOT)
State of Wyoming Department of Employment
Wyoming Division of Vocational Rehabilitation
1100 Herschler Building
Cheyenne, WY 82002
(307) 777-7450

Bibliography

Bandura A. (1986). *Social foundations of thought and action: A social cognitive theory*. Englewood Cliffs, NJ: Prentice–Hall.

Barrett FM. (1984). Sexual implications of multiple sclerosis. In: Simons AF (ed.). *Multiple sclerosis: Psychological and social aspects*. London: William Heinemann Medical Books, Ltd.:54–71.

Bauer HJ, Firnhaber W, Winkler W. (1965). Prognostic criteria in multiple sclerosis. *Annals of the New York Academy of Sciences* 122:542–51.

Baum HM, Rothschild BB. (1981). The incidence and prevalence of reported multiple sclerosis. *Annals of Neurology* 10:420–28.

Berkeley Planning Associates. (1982). *A study of accommodations provided to handicapped employees by federal contractors*. Washington, DC: United States Department of Labor, Employment Standards Administration.

Burnfield A, Burnfield P. (1982). Psychosocial aspects of multiple sclerosis. *Physiotherapy* 68(5):149–50.

Carroll DL, Dorman JD. (1993). *Living well with multiple sclerosis: A guide for patient, caregiver, and family*. New York: Harper Perennial.

Crites J. (1976). A comprehensive model of career development in early adulthood. *Journal of Vocational Behavior* 9:105–18.

Crites J. (1990). *The Career Mastery Inventory*. Boulder, CO: Crites Career Consultants, Inc.

Dawis R. (1987). The Minnesota Theory of Work Adjustment. In: Bolton B (ed.). *Handbook of measurement and evaluation in rehabilitation* (2nd ed.). Baltimore: Paul H. Brookes.

Dawis R, Lofquist L. (1984). *A psychological theory of work adjustment*. Minneapolis: University of Minnesota Press.

Dean G. (1994). World populations with multiple sclerosis. *Neuroepidemiology* 13:1–7.

Devins GM, Edworthy SM, Seland TP, Klein GM, Paul LC, Mandin H. (1993). Differences in illness intrusiveness across rheumatoid arthritis, end–stage renal disease, and multiple sclerosis. *Journal of Nervous and Mental Disease* 181(6):377–81.

Devins GM, Seland TP. (1987). Emotional impact of multiple sclerosis: Recent findings and suggestions for future research. *Psychological Bulletin* 101:363–75.

Devins GM, Seland TP, Klein G, Edworthy SM, Saary MJ. (1993). Stability and determinants of psychosocial well–being in multiple sclerosis. *Rehabilitation Psychology* 38(1):11–26.

Dobren A. (1994). An ecologically oriented conceptual model of vocational rehabilitation of people with acquired midcareer disabilities. *Rehabilitation Counseling Bulletin* 37:215–28.

Duggan EP, Fagan P, Yateman S. (1993). *Employment factors among individuals with multiple sclerosis.* Unpublished manuscript.

DuPont Corporation (1990). *Equal to the task II: DuPont survey of employment of people with disabilities.* Wilmington, DE: E.I. DuPont de Nemours and Company.

Edgley K, Sullivan MJ, Dehoux E. (1991). A survey of multiple sclerosis, part 2: Determinants of employment status. *Canadian Journal of Rehabilitation* 4(3):127–32.

Equal Employment Opportunity Commission (1992). *Technical assistance manual on the employment provisions (Title I) of the Americans with Disabilities Act.* Washington, DC: United States Government Printing Office.

Equal Employment Opportunity Commission & Department of Justice (1991). *The Americans with Disabilities Act handbook.* Washington, DC: United States Government Printing Office.

Falvo D. (1991). *Medical and psychological aspects of chronic illness.* Gaithersburg, MD: Aspen.

Federation Employment and Guidance Services (1957). *Survey of employers' practices and policies in the hiring of physically impaired workers* (HEW Vocational Rehabilitation Grant). New York: Author.

Feldblum, C. (1991). Employment protections. In: West J (ed.). *The Americans with Disabilities Act: From policy to practice.* New York: Milbank Memorial Fund:81–110

Franklin GM, Nelson LM, Filley CM, Heaton RK. (1989). Cognitive loss in multiple sclerosis: Case reports and review of the literature. *Archives of Neurology* 46(2):162–67.

Gecas V. (1989). The social psychology of self–efficacy. *Annual Review of Sociology,* 15:291–316.

Genevie L, Kallos JE, Struenig EL. (1987). Job retention among people with multiple sclerosis. *Journal of Neurologic Rehabilitation* 1:131–35.

Gibbs WE. (1990). Alternative measures to evaluate the impact of vocational rehabilitation services. *Rehabilitation Counseling Bulletin* 34(1):33–43.

Goldberg R. (1992). Toward a model of vocational development of people with disabilities. *Rehabilitation Counseling Bulletin* 35:161–73.

Gordon PA, Lewis MD, Wong D. (1994). Multiple sclerosis: Strategies for rehabilitation counselors. *Journal of Rehabilitation* 60(3):34–38.

Grant I, McDonald WI, Trimble MR, Smith E, Reed R. (1984). Deficient learning and memory in early and middle phases of multiple sclerosis. *Journal of Neurology, Neurosurgery, and Psychiatry* 47:250–55.

Greenwood R, Johnson V, Wilson J, Schriner K. (1988). *RehabMatch*. Fayetteville: Arkansas Research and Training Center in Vocational Rehabilitation.

Gregory RJ, Disler P, Firth S. (1993). Employment and multiple sclerosis in New Zealand. *Journal of Occupational Rehabilitation* 3(2):113–17.

Gross EL, Sinaki M. (1987). Multiple sclerosis. In: Sinaki M (ed.). *Basic clinical rehabilitation medicine*. Philadelphia: B.C. Decker, Inc.:175–81.

Gulick E. (1987). Parsimony and model confirmation of the ADL Self–Care Scale for multiple sclerosis persons. *Nursing Research* 36:278–83.

Gulick E. (1991). Reliability and validity of the Work Assessment Scale for persons with multiple sclerosis. *Nursing Research* 40:107–12.

Gulick EE. (1992). Model for predicting work performance among persons with multiple sclerosis. *Nursing Research* 41(5):266–72.

Gulick E, Bugg A. (1992). Holistic health patterning in multiple sclerosis. *Research in Nursing & Health* 15:175–85.

Gulick EE, Yam M, Touw MM. (1989). Work performance by persons with multiple sclerosis: Conditions that impede or enable the performance of work. *International Journal of Nursing Studies* 26(4):301–11.

Hall H. (1991). *Final Report on the Job Raising Program*. Baltimore: The Development Team, Inc.

Halligan FR, Reznikoff M, Friedman HP, LaRocca NG. (1988). Cognitive dysfunction and change in multiple sclerosis. *Journal of Clinical Psychology* 44(4):540–48.

Hershenson D. (1992). A theoretical model for rehabilitation counseling. *Rehabilitation Counseling Bulletin* 33:268–78.

Houser R, Chace A. (1993). Job satisfaction of people with disabilities placed through a project with industry. *Journal of Rehabilitation* 59(1):45–48.

Johnson G, Johnson R. (1978). *Living with disability: A survey of social services support for multiple sclerosis patients in Scotland.* Unpublished manuscript.

Kalb R, Scheinberg LC (1992). *Multiple sclerosis and the family.* New York: Demos.

Kanfer- F, Goldstein A. (1991). *Helping people change: A textbook of methods.* New York: Pergamon.

Kanungo R. (1982). *Work alienation.* New York: Praeger.

Keniston D. (1995). *SSDI work disincentives and multiple sclerosis: A dignity-of-risk perspective.* Unpublished manuscript.

Ketelaer P, Crijns H, Gausin J, Bouwen R. (1993). *Multiple sclerosis and employment: Synthesis report.* Brussels: Belgian Ministry of Labour and Employment.

Kornblith AB, LaRocca NG, Baum HM. (1986). Employment in individuals with multiple sclerosis. *International Journal of Rehabilitation Research* 9:155–65.

Kosciulek J. (1993). Advances in trait–and–factor theory: A person-environment approach to rehabilitation counseling. *Journal of Applied Rehabilitation Counseling* 24(2):11–14.

Kraft GH. (1981). Multiple sclerosis. In: Stolov WC, Clowers MR (eds.). *Handbook of severe disability.* Washington: United States Department of Education and Rehabilitation Services Administration:111–18.

Kraft GH, Freal JE, Coryell JK. (1986). Disability, disease duration, and rehabilitation service needs in multiple sclerosis: Patient perspectives. *Archives of Physical Medicine and Rehabilitation* 67:164–68.

LaRocca NG. (1995). *Employment and multiple sclerosis.* New York: National Multiple Sclerosis Society.

LaRocca NG, Hall HL. (1990). Multiple sclerosis program: A model for neuropsychiatric disorders. *New Directions for Mental Health Services* 45:49–64.

LaRocca NG, Holland NJ. (1982). Vocational adjustment in multiple sclerosis. *American Rehabilitation*, November, 9–13.

LaRocca NG, Kalb R, Scheinberg LC, Kendall P. (1985). Factors associated with unemployment of patients with multiple sclerosis. *Journal of Chronic Diseases* 38:203–10.

Larsen P. (1990). Psychosocial adjustment in multiple sclerosis. *Rehabilitation Nursing* 15(5):242–47.

Lawry S. (1987). Preface. In: Scheinberg LC, Holland NJ (eds.), *Multiple sclerosis: A guide for patients and their families.* New York: Raven:vii–viii.

Mahoney M. (1995). *The impact of private–pay health care on the employment of people with disabilities.* Unpublished manuscript.

Marsh GG, Ellison GW, Strite C. (1983). Psychosocial and vocational rehabilitation approaches to multiple sclerosis. *Annual Review of Rehabilitation*:3:242–67.

Matkin R. (1995). Private sector rehabilitation. In: *Foundations of the vocational rehabilitation process*. Austin: Pro–Ed:375–98.

Matson RR, Brooks NA. (1977). Adjusting to multiple sclerosis: An exploratory study. *Social Science and Medicine* 11:245–50.

Matthews B. (1985). *Multiple sclerosis: The facts* (2nd ed.). New York: Oxford University Press.

Matthews CB, Cleland CS, Hopper CL. (1970). Neurophysiological patterns in multiple sclerosis. *Diseases of the Nervous System* 31:161–70.

McDaniel C, Gysbers NC. (1992). *Counseling for career development*. San Francisco: Jossey–Bass.

McIntosh–Michaelis SA, Roberts MH, Wilkinson SM, Diamond ID, McLellan DL, Martin JP, Spackman AJ. (1991). The prevalence of cognitive impairment in a community survey of multiple sclerosis. *British Journal of Clinical Psychology* 30:333–48.

Minden SL, Orav J, Reich P. (1987). Depression in multiple sclerosis. *General Hospital Psychiatry* 9:426–34.

Minden SL, Schiffer RB. (1990). Affective disorders in multiple sclerosis: Review and recommendations for clinical research. *Archives of Neurology* 47:98–104.

Mitchell JN. (1981). Multiple sclerosis and the prospects for employment. *Journal of Social and Occupational Medicine* 31:143–58.

Morrissey SP, Miller DH, Kendall BE, Kingsley DPE, Kelly MA, Francis DA, MacManus DG, McDonald WI. (1993). Magnetic resonance imaging as a predictor of multiple sclerosis in patients with mild symptoms. *Brain* 116:135–46.

Mullins JA, Jr, Rumrill PD, Jr, Roessler RT. (in press). The role of the rehabilitation placement consultant in the ADA era. *Work: A Journal of Prevention, Assessment, and Rehabilitation*.

National Multiple Sclerosis Society. (1992). *Compendium of multiple sclerosis information*. New York: Author.

National Multiple Sclerosis Society. (1995). *Today's symptom control . . . Tomorrow's new treatments*. New York: Author.

Neubert DA, Tilson GP, Ianacone RN. (1989). Postsecondary transition needs and employment patterns of individuals with mild disabilities. *Exceptional Children* 55(6):494–500.

Parker R, Szymanski E, Hanley–Maxwell C. (1989). Ecological assessment in supported employment. *Journal of Applied Rehabilitation Counseling* 20(3):26–33.

Peyser JM, Rao SM, LaRocca NG, Kaplan E. (1990). Guidelines for neu-ropsychological research in multiple sclerosis. *Archives of Neurology* 47:94–97.

Poser CM. (1987). Epidemiology and genetics of multiple sclerosis. In: Scheinberg LC, Holland NJ (eds.). *Multiple sclerosis: A guide for patients and their families.* New York: Raven:3–11.

President's Committee on Employment of People with Disabilities (1985). *Employers are asking . . . about the safety of handicapped workers when emergencies occur.* Washington, DC: Government Printing Office.

Rao SM. (1986). Neuropsychology of multiple sclerosis: A critical review. *Journal of Clinical and Experimental Neuropsychology* 8(5):503–42.

Rao SM, Huber SJ, Bornstein RA. (1992). Emotional changes with mul-tiple sclerosis and Parkinson's disease. *Journal of Consulting and Clinical Psychology* 60(3):369–78.

Rao SM, Leo GJ, Ellington L, Nauertz T, Bernardin L, Unverzagt F. (1991). Cognitive dysfunction in multiple sclerosis: Impact on employment and social functioning. *Neurology* 41(5):692–96.

Rao SM, Leo GJ, St. Aubin–Faubert P. (1989). A critical review of the Luria–Nebraska neuropsychological battery literature: VI neurologic cognitive deficit parameters. *International Journal of Clinical Neuropsychology* 11(3):137–42.

Reed CA, Rumrill PD, Jr, Roessler RT, Brown PL, Boen LL. (1994). *The Accommodations Planning Team seminar: An implementation man-ual.* Fayetteville: Arkansas Research and Training Center in Vocational Rehabilitation.

Reingold SC. (1995). *Research directions in multiple sclerosis.* New York: National Multiple Sclerosis Society.

Roessler RT. (1988). A conceptual basis for return–to–work interven-tions. *Rehabilitation Counseling Bulletin* 32:98–107.

Roessler RT. (1995). *The Work Experience Survey.* Fayetteville: Arkansas Research and Training Center in Vocational Rehabilitation.

Roessler RT, Bolton B. (1985). Employment patterns of former voca-tional rehabilitation clients and implications for rehabilitation prac-tice. *Rehabilitation Counseling Bulletin* 28(3):179–87.

Roessler RT, Farley R. (1993). *Return-to-Work: Trainer's manual.* Hot Springs: Arkansas Research and Training Center in Vocational Rehabilitation.

Roessler R, Gottcent J. (1994). The Work Experience Survey: A reason-able accommodation/career development strategy. *Journal of Applied Rehabilitation Counseling* 25(3):16–21.

Roessler R, Rubin S. (1992). *Case management and rehabilitation counseling.* Austin: Pro–Ed.

Roessler RT, Rumrill PD, Jr. (1994a). *Enhancing productivity on your job: The win–win approach to reasonable accommodations.* New York: National Multiple Sclerosis Society.

Roessler RT, Rumrill PD, Jr. (1994b). Strategies for enhancing career maintenance self–efficacy of people with multiple sclerosis. *Journal of Rehabilitation* 60(4):54–59.

Roessler RT, Rumrill PD, Jr. (1995a). The relationship of perceived worksite barriers to job mastery and job satisfaction for employed people with multiple sclerosis. *Rehabilitation Counseling Bulletin* 39(1):2–14.

Roessler RT, Rumrill PD, Jr. (1995b). *Enhancing productivity on your job: The "win–win" approach to reasonable accommodations* (2nd ed.). New York: National Multiple Sclerosis Society.

Roessler RT, Rumrill PD, Jr. (1995c). The Work Experience Survey: A structured interview approach to worksite accommodation planning. *Journal of Job Placement* 11(1):15–19.

Roessler RT, Rumrill PD, Jr, Reed CA. (1995). *The Work Experience Survey (WES) manual: A structured interview for identifying barriers to career maintenance.* Fayetteville, AR: Arkansas Research and Training Center in Vocational Rehabilitation.

Rozin R, Schiff Y, Kahana E, Soffer D. (1975). Vocational status of multiple sclerosis patients in Israel. *Archives of Physical Medicine and Rehabilitation* 56:300–304.

Rubin SE, Roessler RT. (1995). *Foundations of the vocational rehabilitation process.* Austin: Pro–Ed.

Rumrill PD, Jr. (1993). *Increasing the frequency of accommodation requests among persons with multiple sclerosis: A demonstration of the Progressive Request Model.* Unpublished doctoral dissertation, University of Arkansas, Fayetteville.

Rumrill PD, Jr. (1994). The "win–win" approach to Title I of the Americans with Disabilities Act: Preparing college students with disabilities for career–entry placements after graduation. *Journal of Postsecondary Education and Disability* 11(1):15–19.

Rumrill PD, Jr. (in press). Factors associated with unemployment among persons with multiple sclerosis. *Work: A Journal of Prevention, Assessment, and Rehabilitation.*

Rumrill PD, Jr, Battersby JC, Kaleta DA. (in press). Multiple sclerosis: Etiology, incidence, and prevalence. *Work: A Journal of Prevention, Assessment, and Rehabilitation.*

Rumrill PD, Jr, Gordon SE. (1994). Integrated career development services for college students with disabilities: From philosophy to practice. In: Ryan D, McCarthy M (eds.). *NASPA monograph: Disability issues in higher education.* Washington: National Association of Student Personnel Administrators:111–24.

Rumrill PD, Jr, Mullins JA, Jr, Hartshorn CS, Reed CA. (1994). Employing people with disabilities. *Journal of Long–Term Care Administration* 22(1):7–10.

Rumrill PD, Jr, Roessler RT, Boen LL, Brown PL. (1995). The Accommodations Planning Team seminar: Improving prospects for competitive careers for students with disabilities. *College Student Affairs Journal* 14(2):91–101.

Rumrill PD, Jr, Roessler RT, Denny GS. (in press). Increasing confidence in the accommodation request process among persons with multiple sclerosis: A career maintenance self–efficacy intervention. *Journal of Job Placement.*

Rumrill PD, Jr, Roessler RT, Reed CA. (1995). Remove the barriers that hinder performance: Operationalizing Title I of the Americans with Disabilities Act. *Journal of Long–Term Care Administration* 23(2):20–21.

Schapiro RT. (1990). The rehabilitation of multiple sclerosis. *Journal of Neurologic Rehabilitation* 4:215–17.

Schapiro RT. (1994). *Symptom management in multiple sclerosis* (2nd ed.). New York: Demos.

Schletzer VM, Dawis RV, England GW, Lofquist L. (1961). *Attitudinal barriers to employment* (OVR Special Report RD–422). Minneapolis: University of Minnesota Industrial Relations Center.

Schriner KF, Rumrill PD, Parlin R. (1994). Equity in public policy: The political meaning of specialized services for people with disabilities and directions for reform. In: Kiger GG, Hey SC, Linn JG (eds.). *Disability studies: Definitions and diversity.* Rockville, MD: Society for Disability Studies:53–58.

Schriner KF, Rumrill PD, Parlin R. (1995). Rethinking disability policy: Equity in the ADA era and the meaning of specialized services for people with disabilities. *Journal of the Health and Human Services Administration* 17(4):478–500.

Schwartz G, Watson S, Galvin D, Lipoff E. (1989). *The disability management sourcebook.* Washington, DC: Washington Business Group on Health and Institute for Rehabilitation and Disability Management.

Shapiro JP. (1993). *No pity: People with disabilities forging a new civil rights movement.* New York: Random House.

Shontz F. (1975). *The psychological aspects of physical illness and disability.* New York: Macmillan.

Sibley WA. (1996). *Therapeutic claims in multiple sclerosis* (4th ed.). New York: Demos Vermande.

Smith ME, Stone LA, Albert PS, Frank JA, Martin R, Armstrong M, Maloni H, McFarlin DE, McFarland HE. (1994). Multiple sclerosis exacerbations correlate with worsening magnetic resonance imaging scans. *Multiple Sclerosis Quarterly Report* 13(1):6.

Sumner G. (1995). *Project Alliance: A job retention program for employees with chronic illnesses and their employers.* Unpublished manuscript.

Super DE. (1980). A life–span, life–space approach to career development. *Journal of Vocational Behavior* 16:282–98.

Swanson J. (1989). Multiple sclerosis: Update in diagnosis and review of prognostic factors. *Mayo Clinic Proceedings* 64:557–86.

United States Department of Labor (1991). *Dictionary of occupational titles.* Washington, DC: U.S. Government Printing Office.

United States Department of Labor (Annual). *Occupational outlook handbook.* Washington, DC: U.S. Government Printing Office.

United States General Accounting Office (1993). *Vocational rehabilitation: Evidence for federal program's effectiveness is mixed.* Washington, DC: Author.

Waksman BH, Reingold SC, Reynolds WE. (1987). *Research on multiple sclerosis* (3rd ed.). New York: Demos.

Whitaker JN, Williams PH, Layton BA, et al. (1995). Myelin protein in urine of multiple sclerosis patients not linked to new lesions. *Multiple Sclerosis Quarterly Report* 14(1):8–9.

Wineman NM. (1990). Adaptation to multiple sclerosis: The role of social support, functional disability, and perceived uncertainty. *Nursing Research* 39:294–99.

Wolf JK. (1984). Anatomy and function of the nervous system for MSers. In: Wolf JD (ed.), *Mastering multiple sclerosis, A handbook for MSers and families.* Rutland, VT: Academy Books:3–20.

Zunker VG. (1994). *Foundations of career counseling: Applied concepts of life planning.* Pacific Grove, CA: Brooks/Cole Publishing Co.

Index

175